Ra

MW01259133

Beginn... s Raw Feeding
Guide

RAW FEEDING 1⬤1

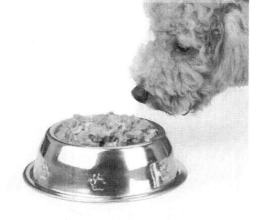

Beginner's
Raw Feeding Guide

Scott J. Marshall II
Certified Raw Dog Food Nutrition Specialist

By Scott Jay Marshall II "Dog Dad"

Raw Dog Food Nutrition Specialist

Legal Information

...well now that we have that awkward stuff out of the way let's move on.

Table Of Contents

Dedications

I could not have put out this book without each and every person in this section. Thank you all, so, so much. You being in my life in one way or another fuels my mission and overwhelms me with a sense of gratitude on a daily basis.

Arianne (My Wife)

What can I say that would even come close to being adequate? You're everything to me. Continuing to support this crazy dream of mine while we worry about whether or not the bills will stay paid, being my biggest cheerleader, calling me on my boulshit, and saying "yes" when I asked the most important question I've ever asked. **"Will you marry me?"**

Wolken & Horus

You cute "little" bastards. Thank you for teaching me what it means to unconditionally love. Without any words at all, you teach me new things about raw feeding, dogs, and myself each and every day.

My Family & Friends

Everyone from my parents, my siblings, my grandparents, my friends, and more have contributed in one way or another to me becoming the person I am today. I cannot thank you enough.

Kimberly Morris Gauthier

My official Raw Feeding BFF (we need to make T-Shirts), I met you at the beginning of 2017 and I truthfully have NO IDEA where I would be without you. It LITERALLY terrifies me think about what things would be like in my life and my business if we hadn't done our first interview on YouTube. You absolutely SMASH (Marvel reference because I know you'll like that) your blog at www.keepthetailwagging.com, you have so much knowledge to share with all of us about you and your dogs, and without a doubt you are the unchallenged social media queen. Could you please stop being so selfish and share the company that produced your clone that helps you put out all that content?

Dewan Bayney

There are very few things I can say in this life with absolute certainty, this is one of them. Without Dewan Bayney, I would not be in business today. End of story. 1 on 1 consultation calls, social media content, moral support and just as importantly, the connections in this world I have made because of you have all made the difference in me being the owner of my own small business. Dewan, you're **THE** man. End of story.

Dale L. Roberts

Dale, you savvy self-publisher you. First you were a dude on Dewan's YouTube channel crushing self-publishing, then a mentor, and finally a dear friend. Thank you for being there through the good times and the bad and never letting me forget that massive action fixes everything. Oh, and for Kelli, "RAWDAWG!!"

Ronny LeJeune

Ronny, it's no secret that you own and operate www.perfectlyrawsome.com and that you hold several certifications. Certified Professional Dog Trainer (CPDT-KA), Canine Conditioning Coach (CCC), and you're constantly going after more. As fantastic as those are, your most important certified is being a (CTB),

Certified Total BadAss. Thanks for reminding me we can't please everyone and that shouldn't bother us. If anything, it should inspire us because we're making enough noise to be noticed.

Rodney Habib

Dude, the impact you've had on this world is incredible. It's nothing short of amazing, truly. Thank you for inspiring me and proving to people like me that even we don't have to have multiple PhDs or anyone's stamp of approval to improve lives. That with a big heart, and a lot more time than we ever anticipated it would take, we can all do our part.

Dr. Karen Becker

Dr. Becker, I thought a lot about what exactly to write here because there would simply be too much for a dedications section of a book if I included everything. I think I've found the best way for me to summarize it.

Thank you for being the veterinary voice this world's pets and pet owners **desperately** needed and deserved.

About The Author

I always find it a little weird to read a lengthy "About The Author" section when I read a book, even if I'm highly interested in the book's subject matter and by extension the author.

With that in mind, I won't bore you.

If you want to learn more about me you can find me on Facebook under "Scott Jay Marshall II", on YouTube at youtube.com/c/dogdad, and at www.dogdadofficial.com & www.rawfeeding101.com.

Foreword

Is it better to feed premade raw or DIY?
Should I choose Prey Model Raw or BARF?
Should I feed my dogs vegetables or no vegetables?
How do I know if the diet is balanced?
What about supplements?
What's golden paste?
Hot and cold foods? What!?!?

Believe it or not, raw feeding is easy. Well, it becomes easier.

In 2013, I turned to the Internet and social media for a crash course in raw feeding and I was immediately overwhelmed. The "professors" contradicted each other, the "faculty" was rude and dismissive, and the "curriculum" didn't make any damn sense. But I kept at it because my dog was thriving on commercial raw and my wallet was screaming that I need to figure out DIY or return to kibble. I couldn't return to dry dog food.

Today, more than 5 years later, Internet searches for "raw feeding" have multiplied because more pet parents want to learn how to feed their dogs a species appropriate diet. To meet that need, we're seeing a rise in content creators, people who are stepping up to teach others how to feed raw to their pets.

That's how I met Scott Jay Marshall II.

I saw and shared one of his YouTube videos and the response I received wasn't what I expected. His loudest critic rattled off a list of why she didn't like him, wrapping up her rant by pointing out that he had A FAT DOG! In her attempt to discredit him, she introduced me to my Raw Feeding BFF and she must have missed that I had A FAT DOG too. Scott and I have been pals ever since.

Learning how to feed your dog a raw food diet comes easy to some people. However, for many of us, it's overwhelming, confusing, and complicated. I don't believe that there will ever be a day when I know everything about feeding a raw diet. Scott has become a valuable resource in the raw feeding community. His passion for raw feeding and helping others comes through in every word. His patience for others is evident in his growing community. And his humility shines through because he is excited to always be learning something new.

If you purchased this book to learn to feed raw, you have taken the first step on a journey to raising healthier pets. You'll enjoy having Scott as your guide on this journey to becoming a raw feeder and you'll find the transition a lot easier than if you were to take the journey alone.

Kimberly Gauthier | Keep the Tail Wagging® | A Novice's Guide to Raw Feeding for Dogs

Why I Wrote This Book

Book V.S. Online

As many of my followers know I created an online video course (Raw Feeding 101 - Learn To Feed Raw) for dog owners that were completely new to this whole "raw feeding thing" that wanted to get their dogs transitioned but had no idea where to start.

So why write a book that for the most part contains the same information as my online course.

YOU, that's why.

To be fair, there will be some people that purchased this book after purchasing the course because they are amazing people that want to support me and my mission.

That being said, online courses and video content overall are not everyone's cup of tea. Maybe they don't like given their credit card information out online (totally understandable) maybe they don't digest information from videos very well, maybe they're just a good ol' fashion bookworm that LOVES to read. It's because of those beautiful bookworms that I created this book.

Don't worry audiobook readers, I didn't forget you which is why I created the audiobook form of this book as well.

My mission is to educate as many dog owners as possible with the end goal of getting as many dogs transitioned to raw as possible. I can't achieve that goal to the best of my abilities by keeping all of the information I have in my course SOLELY online in my course. I needed to deliver it in as many formats and platforms as possible.

So to you beautiful bookworms and busy audiobook-ers, thank you for inspiring me to finally get my butt in gear and product this book.

Do My Part

What do I mean by "Do my part." The year this book was originally written (2018), raw feeding essentially came under mainstream attack. The media, the FDA, kibble manufactures, and so on, all seemed to come out from under a rock at the same time to start slamming fresh foods in every way imaginable.

Doing, in my opinion, biased amounts of uncalled for tests by the FDA on the products from raw pet food manufacturers. Veterinarians plastering anti-raw propaganda while pushing the same brands that sponsored their schools and that now sit on the shelves of their practices. Major pet food manufacturers creating geared towards making the raw feeding movement seem like a dangerous fad that is going to get you and your family sick while harming your dog. Some even going so far as to pay the vet bills for the damage their food caused and/or "replace" your dog, as if you could simply "replace" a dog. It's not a truck.

So, what's my part? My part is to combat this in the ways that I can.

Raw feeding is not any more dangerous than it is to prepare hamburger for a BBQ or a holiday turkey, raw feeders are not a bunch of fad followers that give themselves zero education, and we are certainly not judging kibble and wet food feeders. The VAST majority of us were kibble and wet food feeders at one time or another.

That however is not what the media says because there isn't enough money in it for them.

So how can one dude from northern Utah with a phone for a camera and no Phd to speak of do his part? Content.

Facebook group, Facebook page, Facebook live streams, Facebook posts, Instagram posts, Instagram live streams, YouTube channel, YouTube live streams, the Raw Feeding 101 course, and on and on.

That's another reason that drove me to write this book. One more person sharing their experiences and proving that you don't need a degree in rocket science to feed your dog fresh foods. One more person normalizing the idea of feeding a dog the way nature intended him to be fed.

One more person, creating one more piece of content because one person sharing content can inspire countless dog owners to change the lives of their dogs forever.

Now for what is probably the most important reason I wrote this book, to create real change. The very real change that sprung from Monica's very real and hellacious situation.

Monica's Story…

"Ray Ray has 24-72 hours left at best. He's critical and in renal failure. Take him home, make him comfortable, and don't feed him any processed foods. He can't handle the chemicals in the kibble right now." This paraphrased quote is what Monica heard from her veterinarian. Luckily, that's not where the story ends.

I've decided to include Monica's story in her own words so you can read and feel the real life impact that feeding fresh food creates. Monica has of course consented to this information being shared. The following is a post she made on Facebook 9 months after hearing the heartbreaking statement above.

"WE MADE IT !!!!!!!

This year has been extremely hard on us. We lost our precious Lola the year before to renal failure and here a year later Ray Ray was diagnosed with the same fate. Some would say he's my heart dog, I would tell you he is literally my soul. We ran every lab and test we could and given a grim 24 -72 hour prognosis.

The year before we lost 3 huskies. My heart just wasn't ready to say goodbye. We came very close more times then I can count of having to say goodbye. There have been long long nights where were aren't sure if there is a sunrise yet to be. We fought hard and continue to fight every day for ray ray. We made the commitment to go to an all raw diet for the whole pack. (When you have a pack it's all or nothing and so much easier than trying to sort bowls and foods and food thieves) we dove into the deep end of ocean not even sure if it wasn't too late. Thanks to Courtney McFarlane she led me to Kimberly Morris Gauthier and amazing angel and legend in the raw food movement. I followed her blog , posts open to anything that would give us more time. In meeting Kimberly I was led to the Dog Dad Scott Jay II Marshall, an also equally phenomenal man who also shared loads of knowledge and weekly (every Friday live Q & A) both of these wonderful angels share an abundance of information and help and answer any questions they can and if it's something they don't have the down low on they refer you to someone who does (AMAZING RIGHT?????) with their help, support and the friends I have made in both groups , I am so happy to say that Ray Ray is still here with us! And. Yes at some point he will cross the bridge due to the disease but thanks to Kimberly and Scott we have been given so much more time . We changed their diets and in turn changed their lives. Ray Ray is still here 9 mos later the best gift we could have ever been given. This year I am *so thankful for the new friends I have made , the support I receive in the raw community, the continual education I have learned from both of them.My health ? well it's been touch and go .lots of up and lots of downs. Possible surgery in the future if my lungs are strong. But all in all I think I'm most fortunate, I have a loving son, wonderful husband. Close friends ,dear family and my huskies <3 <3*

That's a lot to be grateful for and I am. I'm hoping 2018 brings me better health, but I'm not picky , if even my lungs got stronger I'd be ecstatic lol. So here's to family, friends, furkids, and health . May 2018 be fruitful for everyone .

I wish you all a very HAPPY NEW YEAR ! ! !
BRING IT 2018 WERE READY <3 <3 <3

Ray Ray made it for approximately one more month after this post was made.

Ray Ray & Monica didn't get one or even 3 more days together, they got **10 MONTHS & 1 DAY**. If someone told you tomorrow that your dog had one day left and by some miracle that turned into ten months, how much would that mean to you?

That's why I wrote this book.

Ten more months of wagging tails when you walk in the front door, ten more months of "kisses" and love, ten more months of not having to say goodbye...

Chapter 1

First Things First

How To Use This Book

So you've purchased the Raw Feeding 101 book and now you need to know exactly HOW to use this book to take you from where you are now, to feeding your dog or dogs a raw diet. I'm going to cover that in this section so let's get started.

Let's first ask "What IS the purpose of this book?" The primary goal of this book is to educate you and get you to a place where you are comfortable with beginning the raw diet and how to continue feeding a raw diet for the rest of your dog or dogs' lives. That being said, I know that some of you may already be raw feeders and simply purchased the book because you want to continue your learning which is of course amazing. Continued learning should be every raw feeder's goal.

With that in mind, there are two ways to use this book.

Method 1 - Going From Start To Finish

The first method of using the book is going to be for a dog owner that is not yet feeding a raw diet and needs a solid foundation before getting started.

With this method you will simply start at the beginning and work your way through the chapters in order starting here in chapter 1 and with the transition instructions occurring in chapter 7.

You can go through all of chapter 7 before starting but don't start your transition in section seven until you have gone through chapters 1 - 6 as well. Remember, the only thing worse than a kibble diet is an unbalanced raw food diet.

The transition chapter of the book is not the end so feel free to either continue on and read ALL of the chapters before your transition, or start the transition when you come to that chapter and simply finish the other chapters at any other time you'd like.

Method 2 - Focused Reading

This second method of using the book is going to be for the dog owner that is already feeding a raw diet but wants to expand their knowledge and learn something new or for someone that just wants to see what this book is all about.

With this method simply through all of the different sections, chapters, and resources and read / use the information at your own pace.

Basically, if you are already feeding raw and fit the type of person I described above, use the book however you would like!

One More Important Note

I consider the book to be broken into two different sections in a different way as well.

There is the necessary information and the additional information. The necessary information is made up of the disclaimer/legal stuff sections, as well as chapters 1-7. The additional information is every chapter AFTER chapter 7. I broke the book up in this way because I wanted my readers to be able to get through the necessary information and transition as quickly as possible.

The additional information is extremely important and should be read without a doubt but is not necessary for the initial transition.

I would however recommend reading the sections on fish oil/omega-3 fatty acids and coconut oil immediately after the initial transition.

They are VERY important supplements, especially omega-3's.

In Conclusion

To recap, if you are a beginner, please read through the book in order from start to finish to ensure that you are receiving a solid foundation of education and knowledge before implementing the raw diet for your dog or dogs.

If you are currently a raw feeder, the world is your oyster and you can read any of the chapters and use any of the resources in any order you would like.

For the beginners, let's move on to the next section. "What Is Raw Feeding & Why Do People Do it?"

What Is Raw Feeding & Why Do People Do It?

What Is It?

Raw feeding or a raw food diet for dogs is all about providing a species appropriate diet, and modeling the natural canine diet. I.E. we're playing copycat with mother nature to the best of our abilities. Makes perfect sense right? There are several different methods of raw feeding that all have their own unique benefits that I will discuss in later in the book.

So WHY do people feed raw foods instead of just scooping kibble out of the bag which would, admittedly, be so MUCH simpler and in many cases cheaper?

Why Do People Do It?

I've been feeding raw now for more than 8 years now and teaching people how in one form or another since 2014. In my experience the "Why people do it" usually boils down to one or a combination of the following three reasons.

Reason 1. New Dog Owners That Demand The Best

There are new dog owners or dog owners to be that are simply looking for the best. In my mind and because you bought this book I have to assume yours as well, raw feeding IS the best option out there when it comes to canine nutrition regardless of which form or model it takes shape in. (More on that later.)

Reason 2. Fear of kibble and other traditional commercial foods.

There has been A LOT of light shed on the pet food industry in the past several years and a lot of people are waking up to the fact that little brown, yellow, and red pellets simply CANNOT be healthy for their dogs and most certainly is not the best option out there.

Reason 3. Damage control.

Many times dog owners come around to raw feeding because they are dealing with one or multiple health problems that can be linked to feeding traditional commercial foods like kibble. These foods have either directly caused, contributed to, or hindered effective treatments of the problem. These problems could include everything from allergic reactions, chronic stomach upset, hair loss, constant itching, and more.

One could argue those are all allergic reactions but that is not where the symptoms end so listing allergic reactions separately felt appropriate. So regardless of which one of these owners the person is, their goals and desires are met when they switch to a raw diet.

They are either doing the absolute best they can because they won't settle for less, they are getting away from the terrifying reality that is the pet food industry and what is being fed to our dogs, or they are looking for a fighting chance at getting rid of the issues that are plaguing their furry best friends and family members.

What To Expect From Raw Feeding & When?

By now, you undoubtedly know that raw feeding is a diet that is far superior to the conventional dry kibble and wet canned foods we have been feeding our dogs for decades BUT do you know what you can expect from raw feeding?

Let's go over a few of the most common benefits and changes people see in their dogs and when they see them.

Changes In Stools

One of the single most common changes in a dog when they are switched to a raw diet is their stools...their poop.

Not only is it one of the most common changes but it is also nearly IMMEDIATE. As long as everything is going well you will see a change in your dog's stool within 24 hours, both frequency AND volume. That means that your dog will go #2 less often, and when they do the amounts will be much smaller and MUCH less stinky in most cases.

As an example, let me tell you a short story. Not too long before the recording of my Raw Feeding 101 2.0 online video course, my wife and I were puppy sitting my in-laws' kibble fed shih-tzu Peyton. We probably puppy sat Peyton for around 5 hours and he went #2 3 different times and produced more stool than either of my 83 lbs+ German Shepherds do in an entire day. That says a lot about how much of the kibble your dog is actually able to digest, absorb, and utilize.

The bottomline is that raw equals a lower overall amount of poop much less often.

Cleaner Teeth

Dental issues are one of the biggest problems plaguing the domestic dog in today's world. According to the AVDC (American Veterinary Dental College) periodontal disease (dental issues) is, *"...the most common clinical condition occurring in adult dogs...".*
I'll go over this in more detail later in the book but raw feeding can act as nature's toothbrush. This means that a raw fed dog on the right diet can LITERALLY be getting an all-natural teeth cleaning at every meal.

The effects of this can be seen in as a little as 24 hours and as long a few weeks. This greatly depends on which raw feeding model you've chosen and the type of recreational chews that you choose. The current state of the dog's teeth also need to be taken into account.

Coat Quality

Every dog owner, especially dog owners that are or know dog groomers, want a dog to not only be healthy, but to look great as well. While many factors go into a dog's cosmetic appearance, all fall second to the dog's coat.

The coat is the majority of what you see on a dog and will immediately stand out if it is having issues. Many of today's kibble and other commercial pet food fed dogs have extremely poor quality coats. Ranging from dry and lackluster in appearance to greasy and undesirable to the touch. Raw feeding can help you there.

One of the members of my raw feeding group community "Raw Feeding 101 - Learn To Feed Raw" on Facebook had this to say about her young female doberman and the impact raw feeding has had on her coat.

"I love how shiny she is, people always compliment her coat and I love telling them it's attributed to her diet."

What can I say, the proof is in the pudding...or should I say puppy?

Typically, this type of change can take several weeks to become fully noticeable or even longer depending on the quality and state of the dog's coat when the transition to raw is made.

Allergy Relief

Allergic reactions caused by commercial diets is running rampant in today's domestic dog. Everything from yeasty ears and paws, skin issues, upset stomachs and more.

A large majority of dogs with these types of reactions that are being caused by their food see dramatic improvement in these issues after the transition if they don't see them go away altogether. The relief from these symptoms will most likely come in stages and take several weeks even months to completely go away as it takes time for the body to rid itself of whatever is causing the issue and then begin repairing the problem.

For example, I have seen many dogs with bald spots caused by allergic reactions to their kibble that immediately started showing improvement after the switch but took months to completely regrow the hair in that area.

Unfortunately, some dogs never did completely regain all the hair in the affected areas but the differences were still quite dramatic.

Longevity

We want our dogs to live longer, healthier, happier lives right? Well raw supporting this longer life is no longer an assumption. We have proof.

A current study ran and established by Thomas Sandberg of longlivingpets.com embarked on a 30 year study in the year 2000. He is nearly 18 years into his 30 year study that is made up of thousands of dogs and cats and has found out 2 very important things.

Number one, that a raw, fresh food diet can double the lifespan of a raw fed dog. DOUBLE, that is absolutely insane. You get to spend twice as many years with your furry best friend just from giving him or her a diet change.

Number two, dogs on this diet show significantly reduced cases of cancer. It's not hard to see why a lack of cancer is going to support longevity.

Obviously, until we build time traveling technology we will never be able to say how long a particular dog would have lived if they had not been put on a raw food diet. That being said, the data polled from the thousands of pets in the Long Living Pets study is enough proof for me.

Energy Returning To Previously Sluggish Dogs

So many of the dogs out there on a commercial dry food diet suffer from one medical issue or another. That may be an allergy, it could be obesity, it could be periodontal issues, joint problems, and the list goes on and on.

Often times a switch to a raw diet eliminates a large number of these issues. This leads to relief of many of the stresses on the body that these issues are causing. This impacts the dog's overall health and well-being in such an extreme way that many dog owners report new vitality and energy in their dogs after the switch.

"It's like a had a whole new dog." or *"It's like my dog was a puppy all over again."* are not uncommon statements to hear from owners after the switch.

As you can see there is a plethora of benefits to raw feeding, in fact there are many more than I listed here.

The bottomline is that with the implementation of a raw food diet, you can create a dramatically higher quality of life for your dog. Period

Alright, on to chapter two!

OVERCOMING MENTAL BARRIERS

Chapter 2

Overcoming Mental Barriers

Significant Others Who Are Weary Of The Switch

Learning how to raw feed your dog or dogs can be hard enough. So what do you do when your significant other disagrees with your desire to start feeding a raw diet to your dog? If you want to start your dog or dogs on a raw diet and your significant other isn't on board for one reason or another, it's obvious to see why that can be a big problem. Especially if you are in a serious relationship.

Well in this section I'm going to give you some simple steps to handle this....hopefully. Nothing is guaranteed with human beings and their opinions. I'm going to break it down into three levels.

Ideally, you'll never have to go to level 3 but let's get into it.

Level 1: Intimately Explaining Your Why & Sharing The Benefits

Sometimes simply sitting down with your significant other and telling them WHY you want to get your dog(s) on a raw diet is enough to tip the scales.

- You WANT your dog to live a happier, healthier, longer life.

- You WANT to spend less on vet visits.

- You WANT to help your dog with their food caused issues.

So on and so on.

The point here is that you are trying to explain exactly where it is that you are coming from and why, seemingly out of nowhere, you want to up and change your dog's diet that has been "working" for as long as it has. Maybe you're getting a puppy that you want to start on raw and your significant other has never heard of or even thought of feeding anything other than traditional dog food. Bottomline you are giving them a look into your point of view.

If your significant other is still hesitant or against the idea it's time to move on to level 2.

Level 2: Addressing Their Specific Concerns With Information & Solutions

So you've gone through your spiel about why you want to feed raw and the benefits associated with this new diet but they are still not ready to get on board, you need to find out why.

Maybe it's because of myths or misinformation they've heard like dogs not being able to eat bones. Another big myth is that raw meat is going to get the dog and the family sick through salmonella, e-coli, etc… Maybe they're concerned about cost which is a completely understandable concern. Maybe they're intimidated by the amount of time it's going to take to learn how to do it.

Of course, they don't need to worry about that one because you bought this book. **wink**

Maybe they're simply afraid. Whether it's being afraid of doing it wrong and hurting the dog, afraid of the time and effort it will take, or any other number of things.

No matter what you do, **DO NOT** belittle their concerns. They respectfully sat through (or at least should have) level 1 when you made your case and you should do the same. Now that you've received that feedback it's time to act on it. Provide some really good information that relieves their concerns caused by the myths and misinformation they have heard. Do a budget and decide exactly what it is that you can afford to spend and exactly how you are going to feed a raw diet while staying within the budget. Figure out how much time it's going to take you how often and commit to a large portion of it, at least in the beginning until they eventually see the light.

The bottomline is you need to respect their concerns and address their concerns whether it be with information or solutions and then revisit the question of whether or not you two are going to do it. Hopefully things stop here but if they don't, it's time to move on to level 3.

Fair warning, level 3 in my opinion is **NOT** for married couples or others in a serious long term relationship.

Level 3: It's Your Dog, Your Call.

awkward pause

Things just got a little uncomfortable didn't they?

Okay, like I said at the end of level 2, I do not recommend using level 3 if you are in a serious relationship. That being said... If you are in a new or casual relationship and your significant other is simply disagreeing with you or giving you a hard time about wanting to feed raw, well I've got one thing to say about that...

...your dog, your call. Period.

If you are in a long term relationship, living with someone, married, etc... then obviously your partner's input really needs to be taken into account. If your relationship doesn't fall into one of those categories then what you feed YOUR dog really isn't any of the other party's business.

I'm personally lucky enough to have never had to deal with this problem. My now wife, then girlfriend was 110% behind my thoughts on raw feeding. We were living together and in a committed relationship so if she would have had objections, the above steps would have been followed.

Feeding a raw diet can be confusing at first and time consuming. So if your significant other isn't with you on it then it just makes the whole thing that much harder. If you find yourself in this situation remember the 3 levels.

Intimately share your thoughts and the benefits of raw feeding, HEAR their concerns and provide education or solutions to those concerns, and really gauge the relationship you are in and whether or not your partner should have a say in what it is that you are feeding your dog.

Criticism From Friends & Family

In this section I want to tell you some simple ways to deal with criticism from friends and family because it WILL happen...unfortunately.

What types of criticism can you expect?

For the vast majority of people, raw feeding is a completely foreign concept so it's not surprising that they have such intense feelings about it. Those feeling might be shock, disgust, confusion, concern, and so on. This could result in a multitude of different criticisms.

They may tell you that you are going to make your dog sick. They may tell you that YOU and the other human members of your family are going to get sick. They might tell you dogs can't eat bones and they are going to choke and die or get some type of intestinal obstruction/blockage from consuming raw bones. They may just be confused and say something like *"I don't get how that is supposed to work?"*

Can we blame them?

They've never heard of dogs eating anything other than traditional dog food on a regular basis their entire life. So how do you deal with these criticisms/questions? You really only have two options.

Option 1: Educate & Converse

Sometimes the people asking these questions or stating these criticisms are simply confused. So IF you are up to the task and you feel like putting out the time and energy (both mental and emotional) you can try and share some information with them and educate them.

Here's why I'm doing this, these are the benefits, I'm trying to solve this issue, etc… Essentially, in a civil and polite manner simply make your case similar to how you would have done in level 1 with your significant other if the need arose.

I find it's best to have a "Go To" statement. Something you've rehearsed ahead of time so you feel confident in what you're saying.

Something like, *"I understand your confusion or misunderstanding and I appreciate your concern. I have done my research and spent a lot of time thinking about this and I've decided it's what's best for my dog(s). If you'd like I can tell you more about it."* is a good example of a "Go To" statement.

Option 2: Disengage

Like I said before, sometimes people are just ignorant to what raw feeding is and with some civil conversation can be "shown the light" and at the very least will respect why it is that you are doing what you're doing.

That being said, there are just as many people out there that are not like that.

Some people just 100% disagree with the idea of raw feeding. This may be because of fear, maybe they've heard of bad experiences, or maybe they simply see that you are doing something different than they are doing and they take it as a judgement on them.

Conversations with these type of people tend to aggressive, judgemental, even malicious on occasion. If you really think you are up to the task then you can attempt to educate and converse like I talked about in option 1. However, if you attempt this or even if you don't and the situation continues to escalate, it's time to remove yourself from that conversation. I'm putting this next sentence in all caps on purpose to drive the point home because I want you to remember it well.
THERE IS NO REASON TO REMAIN IN THAT CONVERSATION.

The bottomline here is that you ARE going to receive comments and criticism from time to time, even from friends and family as sad as that is to say. It's up to you to choose how you deal with that according to the situation and how you feel.

You can either have a conversation and share some information with someone that is seemingly willing to listen, or you can walk away from a negative, toxic conversation.

Get your "Go To" statement ready and be prepared to determine which of the two options you are going to use in any given situation.

Now I'm going to go over how to deal with your veterinarian when it comes to raw feeding...deep breath.

Raw Feeding & Your Veterinarian

Believe it or not, there is a very large number of veterinarians out there that do not support raw feeding and even some that are full blown against and discourage raw feeding. Some of their reasons are good...some not so much. In this section I want to show you how you can handle this unique and important relationship when feeding a raw diet.

Let's get started.

So Why Are Some Vets Against Raw feeding?

Like I mentioned in the opening of this section, there are a ton of reasons that vets disagree with raw feeding and some of them are better than others so let's go over a few just so that you get at least a general idea of where they are coming from.

Reason 1. Old School Thinking

Some vets out there are just simply close minded. For decades they've been trained in a certain way with heavy influences from traditional dog food manufacturers saying their foods are the only safe way to feed a dog and meet their nutritional needs.

Reason 2. They Don't Believe There Is Enough Research Out There

Some vets just don't believe that we have enough science out there to support the validity and safety of a raw food diet.

Reason 3. Lack Of Owner Education

This is one of the only reasons I see eye to eye with vets on. Some vets believe, and are right in believing so, that a percentage of the population interested in feeding a raw diet simply will not do their due diligence and properly educate themselves on how to implement and maintain the diet.

I 100% agree with these veterinarians because in the beginning I was one of those people.
I learned enough to get started on the diet and then stopped learning. This of course was a HUGE mistake that I sincerely hope you will not make after finishing this book.

The fact that you have paid for a book like Raw Feeding 101 shows that you have the drive and passion to NOT be one of these undereducated feeders. Kudos!

Let's move on to some of the different TYPES of veterinarians that you may come across and may already have and the best way to handle the relationship.

Type Of Vet #1: 100% Against Raw Feeding & Refuses To Acknowledge New Information

This is the type of vet that strongly believes in Reason #1. For whatever reason, these types of veterinarians refuse to change their way of thinking or doing things even when scientific evidence is dropped on their desk.

Dealing with these type of veterinarians is going to be extremely difficult.

The best situation you can hope for in this situation is to provide your go to statement that was discussed in a previous section and hope that the vet focuses on issues at hand and doesn't blame every issue the dog has on the raw feeding. If you have your civil discussions and provide your go to statement but continue to receive criticism or the vet refuses to overlook the raw feeding and continues to blame all the dog's issues on it, then I would recommend seeking out a different veterinarian.

Type Of Vet #2: Vet's That Don't Support or Recommend Raw But Do Not Make A Big Deal Out Of It

Yes I know that's a long type name but it is critical to be descriptive here. This type of vet does not support or recommend raw when asked about it. That being said, when they hear about the fact that you feed raw they may make one statement about it, either discouraging or questioning it, but generally leave it alone after that.

This is where our vet fits. Although truth be told, I think we are convincing them on a subconscious level. How can we not be when they constantly tell us how great our dogs look and that the state of their teeth is amazing.

Again this is where our vet fits into the type list. During our first visit they tried to convince us to switch to science diet and I very quickly provided my go to statement and diplomatically got the point across that they were wasting their time on that conversation.

To this vets credit they did send a list of homemade cooked diets for me to check out. Which is of course encouraging because they at least recognize the value of real food in the diet.

All that being said, after that first interaction it has been non eventful when the "What are you feeding" question got brought up and we focused on the reason for the visit. Dealing with this type of vet should be easy enough as long as you are confident in your beliefs in regards to raw feeding, stand your ground, and provide your go to statement, all should be well.

Type Of Vet #3: Vets That Like The Idea Of Raw Feeding But Are Simply Inexperienced

This is the veterinarian that has been paying attention to what has been happening over the past several years with raw feeding WITH an open mind. This vet likes what they are seeing, they are reading the studies that are being published, and are thinking with their hearts, experience, and intuition. Through all of this they are realizing there may be something to this whole raw feeding thing.

Unfortunately they haven't had a lot of experience or direct exposure to it so they have a difficult time with recommendations, etc...

It's my personal belief that as time goes on these vets will seek out training and information on raw feeding and will become better and better at helping out those who have chosen to feed the raw food diet to their dogs.

Dealing with these vets can be a great experience. It's a great experience for you because your vet is behind your decision to feed a raw diet and fully supports you. It's a great experience for your vet because they get more and more real world exposure in their practice to raw feeding and treating raw fed dogs. The similarities, differences, and so on.

If you find one of these vets or have one currently, thank your lucky stars.

Type of Vet #4: Fully Supports Raw & Is Experienced

This is truly the jackpot of veterinarians for raw feeders. They are few and far between but if you find one and become a client of theirs, DON'T let them go.

This type of veterinarian has had experience treating raw fed dogs and are fully aware of the differences between traditionally fed dog health and raw fed dog health. They also will not be blaming random issues on raw feeding like the first two types of vets may.

Dealing with this type of vet SHOULD be an absolutely amazing experience. Just make sure you are just as great of a client. ;)

Some DO NOTs With Vets As A Raw Feeder

DO NOT argue with your vet when it comes to your decision. Give your "Go To" statement and if you can't come to civil, common ground then it's simply time to find another vet.

DO NOT hide the fact that you feed raw from your veterinarian. Telling your vet that you feed raw may be scary but it's a necessary conversation. For one, you'll never know what type of vet you have until you have the conversation. In addition, it is most likely going to come up eventually anyways. Our veterinarians office asks what the dog is eating before we ever see the vet. Lastly, your doctor doesn't like it when you keep secrets about your health and lifestyle. Your vet doesn't like parts of your dog's health and lifestyle being hidden either.

DO NOT criticize veterinarians and demonize them on the internet. This doesn't help anyone. The client - veterinarian relationship and trust has been damaged enough over the last several years. We should be working together as a team with our veterinarians to build and strengthen that trust and relationship. After all you both have the same goal - keeping your dog as happy and healthy as possible for as long as possible.

To summarize this section I want to say this. Your vet should hold a positive place in your mind and your dog's life so if the relationship just isn't working, find a new vet and then move on. That being said, it is your responsibility as the owner to provide your veterinarian with as much information as possible, be as honest as possible, and do your part to make sure that the relationship and trust between you and your vet is strong.

Again, if that is not the case then it is time to seek out a different veterinarian.

Raw Feeding On The Internet

In this section I want to give you a little insight into what to expect on the internet when it comes to raw feeding and how to handle these things to make your life that much easier.

What To Expect & How To Handle It

Raw Feeding Facebook Groups & Other Online Communities

The internet, especially Facebook is full of communities dedicated to sharing information about raw feeding, teaching people how to raw feed, and are open to answering common raw feeding questions. For the most part these communities have some great people in them and can be an abundant resource for continued education type information.

Unfortunately there are also a lot of overly opinionated and down right aggressive individuals in these groups and sometimes even entire groups. If you find yourself being attacked or criticized by individuals within a group, don't be that person that gets in an internet argument. The best thing you can do is contact an admin.

As a group admin myself, I can tell you that the internet comment thread arguments rarely end in anything other than both parties being frustrated and an admin having to calm the situation down. Don't create those situations, simply contact an admin and explain what happened.

If you find yourself in a group where it seems like EVERYONE is aggressive, over opinionated, and quick to attack others it's probably time to find a different raw feeding group. This is especially true if those overly opinionated, aggressive, and quick to attack individuals are the admins. Admins tend to set the tone for groups. So to be frank...if the admins are jerks, a vast majority of their community are probably jerks too.

Sorry, not sorry. It's true.

Also, don't feel surprised or like you are alone if you get kicked out of a raw feeding group on Facebook. Some of the groups out there have some very strict rules and guidelines and provide no warnings to those that don't precisely adhere to their rules and immediately boot those that don't follow those rules. Even if it is a simple matter of disagreeing on feeding models. BARF vs Prey Model for example.

Don't be surprised if you find yourself kicked out of a raw feeding Facebook group, it happens to a lot of people quite often. If you find yourself being kicked out of a group just hold your chin high and find another group, there are TONS of them.

You are welcome to join my raw feeding group "Raw Feeding 101 - Learn To Feed Raw" where we make it our top priority to maintain a positive, supportive environment. You could also check out groups like Raw Feeding University (RFU) that was created and is maintained by Ronny LeJeune, the creator of perfectlyrawsome.com

To wrap things up for this section, just remember that **the internet is the internet.**

There will always be haters, trolls, know it alls, and keyboard rangers out there just waiting for the opportunity to feel superior and put someone else down. DO YOU, be respectful, communicate in a civil manner, don't be one of the trolls, and never be afraid to walk away from a negative situation, person, or group.

101 Different Answers

In this section I want to cover the single most frustrating thing that any new raw feeder will experience.

What does 101 different answers mean?

You read the title of this section so you know that the main concept I will be talking about here is "101 Different Answers", but what am I talking about? This is a term I like to use to describe the response people get when they ask a question about raw feeding on the internet.

The most common place this happens is in raw feeding Facebook groups. Someone will ask a simple question like "How do I know how much heart I can feed?" This is the part where the person that asked the question starts to see "101" different answers and everyone answering the question seems 100% sure that they are right. Thus 101 different answers.

As I'm sure you can imagine, this not only gets extremely frustrating, but causes a TON of confusion for the person asking the question. They are left in a place of panic where they don't know what to do because on top of the 101 different answers, the people that provided the answers are now arguing with each other saying everyone but them is wrong.

Scenarios like this are one of the driving reasons behind putting together this book.

That's not to say that I AM RIGHT and everyone else is wrong. It's quite the opposite actually.

The reason that the concept of "101 different answers" is such a problem is that there very well may be 101 different ways that work. I know, you're ready to pull your hair out as you read this but don't worry, that's what I'm here for.

I say that there could be 101 different ways that is because it's the truth. There is no one perfect diet for humans out there and it's the same with dogs. Some dogs may be allergic to this or that, some may not handle certain proteins well, some need a slower approach than others, so on and so on.

The point is that there are simply too many factors to say that there is one true way to do things and EVERYONE ELSE IS WRONG. That's why the transition steps in chapter 7 of this book try to anticipate as many as the potential "question marks" as possible to help give your dog the best possible shot of having a successful, issue free transition.

How do I pick the right answer?

Sorry but that's kind of a trick question, because there isn't a single "right answer".
That being said there are some things that you can do to make the BEST decision that you can.

Know Where Your Advice Is Coming From

Is the person providing an answer you're considering following, someone with experience like a group admin or someone that you know has been feeding raw for an extended period of time? Have you seen them provide helpful information that has worked out in the past?
Are they recognized as an authority by someone YOU recognize as an authority.

However you do it, if at all possible, try and vet the person you are considering taking advice from. In other words, confirm that they know what they are talking about. There are a lot of well intentioned people out there that could be giving you incorrect advice or advice that isn't going to work for YOUR dog.

This brings us to the second thing you should do before you implement anyone's advice when it comes to feeding your dog. Knowing YOUR dog.

Knowing YOUR Dog

If you have had your dog for a long time you undoubtedly know things about them that others simply don't and couldn't without spending the same amount of time with them that you have.

Maybe your dog has never adjusted to new foods well, even when switching from one kibble "formula" like chicken and rice to the same chicken & rice "formula" from a different brand. Maybe you have always had to introduce new foods slowly to prevent your dog from experiencing digestive upset. Knowing these kinds of things about your dog's general disposition or traits is going to be critical when deciding what advice to take and act on from online suggestions.

For example, (you'll learn about this more later) I recommend a slow transition and some people recommend a "balanced from the get go" transition. Like I had stated earlier with different things working for different dogs, both of these methods have the potential to be successful. That being said, if you KNOW that your dog has never responded well to food changes then the "balanced from the start" approach, in my personal opinion, holds a lot of potential for problems for YOUR dog.

The reason I say that is because in this example we are dealing with a dog that has always needed to be introduced to foods slowly to prevent or at least minimize negative reactions.
With that in mind, we would want to model that with raw feeding. Slow approaches with one new thing at a time until they adjust and

then move onto the next thing. Even though the dog is being switched to a superior, species appropriate diet, the dog is probably going to continue to respond better to slow changes in their diet. You can change a lot of things in a major and positive way with raw feeding but some things like sensitivity to changes are just plain hard wired into some dogs.

Armed with the "Know YOUR dog." mentality, you can use your best judgement and knowledge of your dog to choose advice that just seems like it would be the best fit for your dog.

Trial & Error

Sometimes, no matter how well we vet advice and sources, no matter how hard we try to choose methods and solutions that we think are going to work best for our dogs, sometimes things just don't work out.

In these situations, you just need to keep trying.

I wish it was a more magical answer but that's the truth. It's like some of the visits you and I have when we go to the doctor. Your doctor will tell you, "Let's give this a shot and come back in 2 weeks if it doesn't get better." Humans and other animals are complicated biological machines and there are definitive answers for very few things.

Bottomline, there is no one perfect answer to every question or problem when it comes to raw feeding and if you ask for advice you WILL get 101 different answers. It's up to you to use everything at your disposal to do your best to make the best possible decisions for YOUR dog.

Marketing Generated Fears

I want to get straight to the point in this section as it pricks a particular nerve with myself and countless other raw feeding / fresh food advocates out there.

For more than half of a century the pet food industry has been using clever and well funded marketing to tell us that they are providing the best possible diet for our dogs.

- Dog foods specifically formulated for this issue and that.
- Dog foods specifically formulated for big dogs and small dogs.
- Dog foods even specifically formulated for specific breeds.

For that same half a century they have been using that same well funded marketing to tell us that their products are the only way to provide a balanced diet. Telling us that anything other than "expertly formulated" traditional dog foods in a bag or tin can is dangerous.

In more recent history these same companies have been flooding our vet offices with pamphlets and short reads on the dangers of raw meats, bones, fresh eggs, and so on, preying on the fear of ignorant, loving dog owners who simply want the best for their furry family members.

Approximate to the time this section was written, one of these companies even had the audacity to label their kibble as "biologically appropriate" as if to claim that in some parallel universe canines used to hunt bags of kibble for sustenance.

I don't tell you these things to complain or to call out those that feed kibble. The vast majority of the public simply doesn't know of anything other way to feed their dogs than with kibble and canned food because of these very successful marketing campaigns I just described and those loving pet parents are simply doing what they believe is best.

I tell you these things so that you are aware that they indeed have been extremely successful in their clever marketing. They have so many people so afraid to do anything other than what this marketing has taught them that some people will never switch to raw simply out of fear and that truly breaks my heart.

Most importantly, I tell you this because as a new raw feeder, there WILL be times where some of the things you learn will challenge what these marketing campaigns have programmed into the public all these years.

When this happens you need to find strength in the fact that more and more science is coming out everyday to prove that raw feeding IS the superior diet. You also need to find confidence and comfort in the fact that THOUSANDS AND THOUSANDS AND THOUSANDS of dog owners and their countless numbers of dogs are following this type of diet RIGHT NOW as you read these words and are leading happy, healthy, thriving lives.

Some of them, like my friend Monica, even got MORE TIME with their dogs before they crossed the rainbow bridge because of raw feeding.

With a little time, the help of this book, and a little courage, you will be on your way to experiencing the same benefits and seeing just how doable raw feeding is for the average dog owner.

Things Happen To Everyone - Don't Overreact

This is going to be a really short section because I only have one point to make but it's a really important point and therefore warrants it's own section.

So what is this one point that I want to make? It's really, really simple.

Things happen to everyone, period.

Now there is a really good chance that you will get through your transition without any major issues. Your dog will react well to the slow transition I am going to talk about later in the book, they'll accept new proteins, organs, bone, and so on and you may even get what seems like a whole new dog with renewed vigor, energy, and vitality.

That being said, things happen, and they happen to everyone at some point or another.
The important thing to remember is DON'T OVERREACT.

Diarrhea and vomit are a perfect example.

If you get through the entire, (hopefully long) life of a dog and they never once throw up or have a bout of diarrhea then I would love to hear where you bought your alien engineered super dog from because I want one.

YOU

I've helped over 28,000 people in their raw feeding journey in one way or another. Some directly, some indirectly, some through my course, some through this book, some through my online coaching, some through my raw feeding FB group, so on and so on.

Without a doubt there has been one, single most common issue for people that prevents them from making the switch or at the very least keeps them in limbo land for a lot longer than they needed to be there. By limbo land I mean that they KNOW raw feeding is superior to commercial dog food, and they have done a ton of research but are still feeding commercial dog food.

This extremely common problem is the person themselves. If we were talking about your situation, it would be, drumroll please....YOU. That's right, YOU.

Right now you are probably thinking, "Hey man, back off." Relax, relax. I don't mean that YOU are necessarily a problem, more that you may get in your own way if you're not careful. It's not really your fault and you definitely wouldn't be alone. Like I said, this is THE MOST common problem that there is which really surprises people until someone like me points it out to them.

Chapter 3

Myths, Models, & More

Raw Feeding Myths

Unfortunately there are A LOT of myths surrounding raw feeding. Even more unfortunate is that many of these myths prevent a lot of people from making the switch and essentially scare them away. That's why in this section I want to address some of the most common myths.

Let's get started!

Raw Feeding Will Make Your Dog Aggressive

`The theory behind raw feeding making dogs aggressive comes from people believing that raw food gives the dogs a taste for flesh and blood. Because we as humans and our other pets are also made of flesh and blood, some people think that raw feeding will essentially make them want to come after us for that next "taste".

While I am not an animal behaviorist I can say that I have never come across a case where a dog that was not aggressive suddenly started turning on the family and fellow animals after being switched. Nor have I read any studies that have shown even one dog that was evaluated and deemed non-aggressive before the switch to a raw food diet by an animal behavior specialist that suddenly became aggressive after the switch.

I personally feel like this is just a case of people not identifying a particular behavior as aggressive before the switch and then all of the sudden "noticing" that it is actually aggressive behavior because they are paying more attention after the switch.

This again is just my personal opinion, it is a very solid NO, raw feeding does not turn non-aggressive dogs aggressive.

That being said…raw feeding MAY cause your dog to start portraying "resource guarding behavior". Here's the deal.

For those that don't know what resource guarding is, it's basically the dog "guarding" or not allowing someone to come near an item or take an item from them. Think about the toddler that turns away from you and screams after you tell them to give you their favorite toy because they're going to time out. Essentially that's resource guarding, only your "toddler" has a mouth full of sharp teeth and may do more than scream if pushed far enough.

This will generally happen when you are feeding whole foods, rec chews, or other food items that the dog isn't going to consume all at once and at some point you'll have to take it away. The fact that your dog has chewed on that item for so long has made it a very "high value" item that they may REALLY not want to give up.

IF this behavior manifests there are a number of ways you can manage it like "trading" the high value food item for another high value food item but if this behavior manifests I would recommend contacting a qualified dog trainer that can teach you in person how best to manage the behavior.

A big thanks to certified dog trainer, Ronny LeJeune of www.perfectlyrawsome.com that taught me about this relationship between raw feeding and resource guarding in an interview I did with her on my YouTube channel, "Dog Dad". If you'd like to watch the full interview simply search "Ronny LeJeune Dog Dad" in the search bar on YouTube.

Bones Splinter & Kill Dogs

This is another one that I've heard countless times. People believe that chicken bones, rib bones, etc...split into shards when they are eaten and because of this the dog is going to die of an obstruction or puncture to the digestive system. While things do happen in extremely rare cases, this is for the most part, false.

This myth started from a truly dangerous practice though, feeding COOKED bones. You see raw bones and cooked bones are VERY different. Raw bones are packed full of moisture, provide an abundance of tooth cleaning benefits, exercise the jaw and shoulders, and break into small & pliable pieces that are easily digested in the digestive system of a healthy dog.

Cooked bones on the other hand couldn't be any more different.

When bones are cooked, moisture is slowly pulled out of the bones leaving them dry. These dry bones EASILY splinter when they are chewed and often times DO splinter into sharp points and edges and can cause real, sometimes life threatening punctures and obstructions. More importantly, they are not digested in the same way leading to the same problems. Nature never intended canines to eat cooked bones and you should never, ever, ever feed them.

Dogs Will Get Sick From Salmonella & E-Coli

This is yet another widely talked about rumor that is just plain not true as long as your dog has a healthy, properly functioning immune system.

Reason 1 - Not all meat is contaminated with Salmonella or E-coli. These are bacterial infections that have to be introduced from an outside source. This leads us to reason #2

Reason #2 - We are able to largely control the quality of meat that we provide our dogs and as long as that food is coming from a trusted source then there is very little chance that the meat is heavily contaminated by these bacterial infections. If they DO happen to have some level of contamination then...well that's #3.

Reason #3 - Nature designed dogs to eat a raw diet. We won't even go into the biomechanics of how dogs are designed specifically to hunt and eat prey animals. Instead let's focus on the digestive system.

Dogs use their clearly carnivore style mouths and teeth to rip, tear and shred flesh as well as crunching through bones, ligaments, cartilage, and more. Then the food goes to the stomach which is HIGHLY acidic where these bacterial infections would have an EXTREMELY hard time surviving. This is one reason why minor levels of contamination combined with proper sanitation often to lead to zero issues. This is why sourcing from safe and trusted sources is so important. The food then leaves the stomach and enters the intestines where digestion is completed, ultimately leaving through the anus.

This entire digestive system is considered an overall "short" or "quick" system. This expedited process of digestion makes it extremely difficult for bacterial infections to not only survive, but be in the system long enough to replicate and cause issues.

Bottomline, your dog was built to eat raw foods and has the protection and digestive system to handle it as long as they are healthy and have properly functioning immune systems.

You & Your Family Will Get Sick

This is an understandable concern. Even the most avid dog lover that is hell bent on providing their dog a raw diet will have bells go off when they hear myths about people and their families getting sick after the switch. This can all be prevented with simple, common sense sanitation steps that we will go into in detail later in the book.

The short version is that if you aren't letting your dog give you kisses right after dinner time, you are cleaning up your surfaces, dishes, utensils, knives, etc...that you are using with your dogs raw food, and you are thoroughly washing your hands with soap and warm water, then all will most likely be well.

As I have previously stated I have helped over 28,000 people with raw feeding in one way or another and I've only heard of one story where raw dog food was the source of someone getting sick.

Well...sort of.

This person who shall rename nameless had a few adult beverages and decided to separate raw dog food and cook dinner at the same time...can you see where this is going?

Long story short, they dipped their finger in dinner to give it a taste with their chicken juice covered finger...I think you can guess what happened next.

So you COULD say that raw food got this person sick but I think it would be more accurate to blame the beverages and poor decision making.

When all is said and done, there is a lot of misinformation out there so I hope that this section cleared some of those up. Raw food does NOT make a docile dog aggressive.
Bones DO NOT automatically kill dogs, at least not raw ones. Your dog is not going to get sick as long as they have a healthy immune system and eat high quality foods provided by you
and simple household sanitation practices are going to prevent you and your human family members from ever getting sick.

That is...unless you throw back a few cold ones and decide to sample dinner with chicken juice drenched fingers....

...please don't do that...pretty please?

Raw Feeding Models & Choosing One For Your Dog

It may surprise you to learn that there is more than ONE way to raw feed your dog or as we like to call them, "models". Like anything else there are people out there that you could call "purists" that say there is only "one true" way to feed a raw diet. Like most "purists" of any kind out there, they will try and sway you to their side of the fence and it's your choice to decide if that side of the fence looks better.

What I'm going to do in this section is provide you with some very black and white information about what describes each of the different models of raw feeding. I also want to provide some tips on choosing which one is right for you and your dog.

What Are The Different Models Of Raw Feeding?

Model #1 Premade

Premade is exactly what it sounds like. Instead of gathering individual pieces of the diet and assembling them yourself (DIY), premade manufacturers do this work ahead of time for you. Premade raw comes in a variety of "flavors", not really flavors but different base proteins like chicken, beef, venison, etc... This is of course a very simplified explanation of the process but essentially the animal is processed and turned into frozen patties, similar to what you see hamburger and turkey burger patties being made into that you buy at the grocery store for your Saturday afternoon summer BBQs. While Formulas are often different from company to company, most of these blends contain meat, bone, liver, and other organs.

Like I said though, this is often very different. For example, many companies do not include bones of any kind and some may or may not add fruits and vegetables. Some companies do not include any type of non-liver organ (the other 5%). Again, each company is a little different.

Premades often one of the first steps into feeding a raw diet that people take because it eases a lot of their worries about providing a balanced diet. That being said I do have to say that I can't agree with a diet completely void of bones and non-liver organ so check your sources carefully.

Some people feel that this is not something that should be used as an entire diet because it does not provide any meaty bones for the animal to chew which exercises the jaw, shoulder muscles, neck muscles, and cleans the teeth.

You won't hear me take a side on many things in the raw feeding world because there are so many mix and match ways to do things and there are few wrong and right answers but in this case I would have to recommend that if you do choose to go with the premade route that you provide some type of meaty bones a couple times a week to ensure your dog is getting the benefits listed above.

Model #2 Prey Model

The next type of raw feeding that I am going to cover is what is called the prey model diet. For newbies this model is often confused with and referred to as the "Whole Prey Diet" but they are two separate methods in a lot of ways. I will address the Whole Prey model later in this section.

People that choose to feed a raw diet in the form of the prey model diet generally believe and feel that dogs are 100% carnivores and should be fed nothing that did not come from an animal. They feed meat, bones, raw meaty bones, organs, and so on. Basically anything that was once part of a living creature. Whether that was a fish, a bird, a cow, elk, kangaroo, ostrich, emu, the list goes on and on. If it was moving around and breathing at some point it's fair game with few exceptions.

Again, GENERALLY, those that feed this style of feeding feel that fruits and vegetables do not belong in a dog's diet and therefore do not feed it in any amount. They feel that not only is it unnecessary but is in some cases, damaging to the dog. Typically these feeders also tend to stay away from any type of supplementation like fish oil and tend to opt for whole food supplementation. I.E. whole fish instead of fish oil.

Now that you have a sense of what a prey model diet is and what it looks like let's take a look at the whole prey model.

Model #3 Whole Prey

Whole prey isn't going to require a lot of explanation because it is extremely similar to the prey model diet.

The whole prey diet is essentially the prey model diet but instead of feeding parts of an animal like pork ribs with rabbit meat, beef kidney and chick liver… like you may see in the bowl of a prey model fed dog, whole prey feeders feed the entire animal...intact for the most part.

As an example, they might feed a whole rabbit or a whole chicken, maybe a quail and so on. There are also circumstances where very large portions of an animal are fed like pig heads, cow, elk, and venison legs.

The stance behind this for those that choose this model of feeding is you are taking yet another step towards modeling the diet of ancestral dogs. So they are eating fur, feathers, skulls, brains, and so on.

For some, this is the hardest model to feed for a lot of reasons. For one, you are seeing an entire animal instead of pieces that you're used to seeing in the grocery store. This may cause some to more empathy for the animal being fed. Maybe you're a vegetarian or vegan and feeding meat is already hard enough for you without having to see a whole animal complete with a face and fur. Another reason this is a difficult way to feed is that some dogs get confused if they weren't introduced to whole prey at an early age. They see an animal there and aren't sure what to do with it.

If they are pet dogs they've most likely been highly encouraged to not bite, attack, let alone eat other animals so they often sniff and look back at you with a look that says, "What am I supposed to do with this? Where's dinner?"

Possibly the biggest reason this type is more difficult is because it's significantly harder to source whole animals. Most people that desire to feed a whole prey diet end up feeding a hybrid diet which we will talk about in this section as well.

Time to move on to the next diet model which is called B.A.R.F..
Yes you heard me right, B.A.R.F..
Don't worry, it's just an acronym.

Model #4 B.A.R.F.

B.A.R.F.. Yes I know it doesn't exactly sound appealing but like I said B.A.R.F. is an acronym. Some say biologically appropriate raw feeding, some say say food, some say bones and raw food, but I think you get the point. It's a way of feeding that is biologically appropriate and is raw.

To set up a framework for B.A.R.F. to illustrate what it is I want you to think about the prey model diet and you have a large portion of what B.A.R.F. is. As far as animal content goes, B.A.R.F. is for all major purposes identical to the prey model diet. The main difference between the two is that B.A.R.F. model feeders also feed produce like fruits and vegetables. Sometimes the fruits and vegetables are pureed before feeding, sometimes they are boiled and pureed. This is done in an attempt to make the food more bioavailable.

In addition to fruits and vegetables B.A.R.F. feeders often times will feed supplements where a prey model feeder would opt for whole food instead. This could include things like glucosamine chondroitin or other items like coconut oil and fish oil. B.A.R.F. feeders generally feel that there are holes in the nutritional needs of dogs that can't be solved with animal parts alone. This is where the vegetables, fruit, and supplements come into the equation.

In short, B.A.R.F. is prey model with fruits and vegetables with some optional add ons like supplements and oils.

Model #5 Hybrid Diets

No, I'm not talking about feeding genetically modified hybrid animals like a rabbichicken or turkeduck. I mean mixing and matching the diets to meet individual needs. This by the way is the section of the book that would upset some of the purists that I mentioned earlier.

Someone may identify as a prey model feeder that occasionally feeds fruits and vegetables.
Maybe another person identifies as a whole prey diet feeder but was unable to source whole prey at the moment and so they feed more of a prey model type diet until they are able to find a reliable, consistent source of whole prey again. Maybe, someone chose to go the premade route but is feeding a premade that requires other things being added into the diet like bone content or a non-liver organ source. I mentioned earlier that some premades do not meet ALL of the nutritional needs like bone and non-liver organs so these things can be added in addition to the premade ground foods.

As a personal example, I identify as a hybrid feeder. While I do mainly provide what appears to be a prey model diet, I do add things to the diet that purists would banish me from prey model land for. I occasionally give a whole carrot. or slices of things like cucumber JUST BECAUSE.

I also on a regular basis add fish oil to my dogs diet because one of them simply cannot tolerate whole fish. Additionally, I provide other supplements including, but not limited to golden paste, bone broth, kefir, PhAdjust. I also have plans to add fermented vegetables to my dogs' diets in the very near future for the microbiome/immune benefits they provide.

In the end there is no wrong answer, but you do need to make a choice on what type of diet you want to feed, especially in the beginning so you have a sort of blueprint or template to follow.

How To Decide Which Is Best For You & Your Dog(s)?

What type should you feed? I have no idea….

Now you may be thinking "Wait a minute, I bought this book so I could be told exactly what to do." Well yes you did, but like I said in the last section on hybrid diets, there is no wrong answer.
You want to feed whole prey model, go for it. Do you want to feed prey model, awesome. Do you want to feed BARF, fantastic. Do you want to feed premade, perfect.

There is no wrong or right answer.

Don't EVER let someone in a Face group, forum, in real life, or otherwise bully you into one way or the other or tell you the choice you made was the wrong one because they're just wrong.
I'll say it one more time cause I really want you to instill this as a belief and fact in your head.

THERE IS NO WRONG ANSWER.

Just by making the choice to feed some sort of species appropriate diet, complete with fresh, raw, whole foods has put you leagues ahead of the vast majority of dog owners when it comes to nutritional health.

The model that you choose is the perfect choice. That being said, you will most likely transition into somewhat of a hybrid diet as time goes by anyways. Almost everyone does.

THERE IS NO WRONG ANSWER. Pick what fits your preferences, lifestyle, and dog's needs and run with it. You can always adjust, modify, and hybridize as you go. In fact I can confidently say that you should ALWAYS be looking for areas to tweak and improve your dog's diet for their benefit and yours. Never get stuck in one lane of thinking. There is way too much information coming out for us to close the blinds to new information that allow us to do an even better job of providing our dogs with optimum nutrition.

The "Secret Formula" 80/10/5/5

In this section I want to talk about the "Secret Formula" for raw feeding. If you've ever spent any time in raw feeding Facebook groups or done any other research online you've probably seen references to this. That "Secret Formula" is 80/10/10. It doesn't seem like anything special right? Well it's super important so let's talk about what it is, what it represents, and whether or not it's perfect for everyone.

What Does The 80/10/10 Represent?

This is actually really simple. They represent percentages of certain things in the dog's diet. 80% muscle meat, 10% bone and 10% organs including liver and other secreting organs.
That essentially is the blueprint for the beginning of your dog's raw diet.

Now Wait A Minute, Is It 80/10/10 or 80/10/5/5?

In any previous digging you may or may not have done prior to buying this book you may have also come across 80/10/5/5. So what's the difference and which one is right? Well the answer is both. One is just a deeper look into the organs portion of the formula. When we look deeper, the 10% organ can be more accurately expressed as 5% liver, 5% non-liver organ. Things like spleen, kidney, testicles, ovaries, sweetbreads, and so on are part of the non-liver 5% organs. I prefer referring to and teaching it as 80/10/5/5 because it seems to help beginners remember that liver should not be the only organ that should be fed.

Where Did The 80/10/5/5 From?

No one knows. Really. In 2018, my "Raw Feeding B.F.F." Kimberly Morris Gauthier of www.keepthetailwagging.com hosted the first annual "National Raw Feeding Week" where she interviewed and spoke with several industry leaders. The common questions she asked everyone was "Where did 80/10/10 come from?" The overwhelming response, paraphrasing of course, (myself included) was "I don't know."

My best guess, as well as the guess of many others is that at some point or another someone tried to represent the approximate amount of the items represented in the 80/10/10 formula that would be found in a prey animal like a rabbit. That is to say that approximately 80% of the animal would have been meat and meaty tissues, 10% of the animal would have been bones, and 10% would have been organs.

After years and years of these being repeated in Facebook groups, before that Yahoo groups, and before that online forums, this formula became "law" if you will. To reiterate, no one knows exactly where this came from. I would love to see proof of the origin of this and/or the original post in whatever forum it showed up in but that is unlikely to happen.
For now, we use it as a guideline to help beginning and newbie raw feeders have a blueprint of sorts to get started on.

So with these measurements being so approximate and it's origin being so unknown, does the 80/10/10 or 80/10/5/5 work for all dogs?

80/10/5/5, does it work for everyone?

Yes and no. I know, I know I'll explain I promise. Yes because this is the most common starting point for raw feeders across the world and there is good reason for it, it works. This again is an approximate measurement of what we are looking for in the beginning of the diet. With this in mind, most dogs do fairly well at this approximate amount and with some self-education and minimal tweaking it can be modified to suit your dog's needs in the long term.

For example, I feed 3 oz of bone when I SHOULD, according to the formula be feeding 2.2 oz of bone because of learned through time and observation that my dogs' poop becomes soft if they don't have that little bit extra.

(More on soft and solid poops later in the book)

No because there is also a large number of raw feeders that have had to make minor to drastic changes to these percentages.

For example, one of the first students of my online course "Raw Feeding 101 - Learn To Feed Raw" had a dog that was struggling with solid poops. After hours of free back and forth sessions with me she decided to see a holistic, raw supporting and experienced veterinarian and had to bring their dog to 24% to stabilize and get solid poops. After that the percentage was slowly lowered over time but the point is that each dog is different and while the 80/10/5/5 works for most dogs, there are dogs out there that will need minor to drastic modifications to these percentages.

So there you have it, the "Secret Formula" that you may or may not have seen talked about so much on the web.

The 2 most important things to take away from this is:
- What the 80/10/5/5 represents.
  - (80% muscle meat - 10% bone - 5% liver - 5% non-liver organ)
- That the secret formula is a great starting point but will need to be modified from one dog to another. Remember, dogs are individuals and you need to do what is ideal for YOUR dog.

What The Poo Tells You

In this section I want to cover a topic that no one wants to talk about, unless you get into a raw feeding group on Facebook and then it seems like it's half of what everyone is talking about, and for good reason. What I want to talk about in this section is your dog's poop and what it can tell you as a raw feeder.

Let's do this!

First of all, let's talk about what's going to change with your dog's poop after the switch and as far as poop conversations go I think you'll be pleasantly surprised with what you can expect to see.

Change #1 - Less Stink

Yup, you read that right, it stinks less. Almost every person that successfully transitions their dog or dogs to a raw diet reports poops that are significantly less...fragrant than it was when they were feeding their dog traditional dog food like kibble or canned food.

Change #2 - Less Poop

Once again, yes you read that right. That brown bomb your precious labrador leaves on the lawn is going to dramatically reduce in size. To put in it's most basic terms, your dog is eating REAL FOOD and not a bunch of cra...stuff found in traditional dog food that your dog's body simply wasn't using.

For example, **TMI WARNING** my German Shepherds on average produce 6"x 1" ahem..."logs" 1-2 times a day. That's it. There are of course exceptions if they had an excessive amount of training treats or extra food but that is the average and these 2 dogs are 83 lbs and 100 lbs.

Change #3 - Less Frequent Poops

One thing that I see time and time again in my Raw Feeding 101 Facebook group is new feeders becoming suddenly concerned because "I think my dog is constipated, he's only gone #2 once in the last 24 hours."

This is completely normal.

Like I referenced earlier, raw feeding is providing your dog's body with REAL FOOD and they are utilizing more of what they consume which results in less poop. These smaller amounts of poop also translate into less frequent poops.
I was recently dog sitting my in-laws' shih tzu and in a 5 hour period he went #2 **5 TIMES!** Each time producing just as much if not more than my German Shepherds do on average in an entire day. It was a great reminder of how lucky I am as a raw feeder when it comes to poop pick up time.

Basically, when you transition your dog to raw feeding you are going to have smaller poops to pick up that stink less and happen less often.

Raw feeding for the win!

Now let's talk about what you are looking for when it comes to your dog's poop and what you don't want to see.

What are you ideally looking for?

The "holy grail" of raw fed dogs is chocolate colored, solid poops. The kind that you can easily lift off grass and you don't leave half of it behind when you try and pull it away.

There can be a slight change in color depending on what proteins they have been eating. Typically red meats cause darker colored poops and white meats, the opposite but your dog may experience little to no change from one protein to the next.

This type of poop is telling you that you for the most part that you have a balanced diet. You're not feeding too much bone, you're not feeding too much liver or organ, and all is well in the world and most likely nothing drastic should be changed.

There are however two common problem poops that typically signal an imbalance in the diet that you can easily change.

Common Problem Poop #1 - Crumbly Poops

This is the type of poop that literally falls apart and disappears into the grass when you try to pick it up. (Aren't you loving all these poop visuals?) Sometimes this can be accompanied by a slightly lighter color of poop but not always.

This type of poop is telling you that there is too much calcium in your dog's diet. Bone is full of calcium that is great and necessary for our dogs but too much is not good. To fix this problem, you can drop your bone content a little bit at a time until you reach the holy grail poop. Now a random, isolated occurrence of crumbly poop is not the end of the world and doesn't necessarily warrant a change in diet but if you are seeing this type of poop several days in a row then it's time to modify the diet by lowering the bone content in your dogs' meals.

Common Problem Poop #2 - Goo Poo

Goo poo or the more "adult" way of saying it, soft stools, is the type of poop that you just CAN'T seem to pick up. You try and try but it just seems like you are smearing it all over the grass and you are having to pull up grass or get the hose to avoid leaving A LOT of it behind.

This type of poop is reporting the exact opposite of what crumbly poops was telling us. This type of poop is often times telling us that there is not ENOUGH bone/calcium in the dog's diet.

To fix this problem you can increase your dog's bone content little by little until you achieve firm, easy to pick up, holy grail poops. Just like crumbly poops, a single occurrence of goo poo should not be cause for concern and should not prompt you into overhauling your dog's diet but if it is a consistent issue it's time to increase that bone content until you get what you're looking for.

New feeders often see a problem with this in the beginning and may have to provide a temporarily higher amount of bone until the dog adjusts to raw feeding. After which the bone should slowly be decreased until you again reach your desired results. My student I referenced earlier is a perfect example of this.

Raw Food Sources

In this section I want to cover something that trips a lot of people up and is one of the most common reasons curious people never start feeding a raw diet. "Where do I get my raw food from?" Where to source your food from comes down to 2 categories, consistent sources and inconsistent sources. Let's look at exactly what qualifies for each of these categories.

What Is A Consistent Source?

Consistent sources are sources that you can get food from on a regular basis that are almost always available. In other words, you know where it is and can get food from there whenever you need to.

Some consistent food sources include:
- Local Grocery Store
- Ethnic Markets/Stores
- Online Sellers
- Local Raw Pet Food Stores
- Butcher (Half & Half)

Grocery Stores

Grocery stores an amazing and almost necessary consistent resource for some people. You won't find as much variety here but it is an extremely reliable place to source from because short of going out of business, the grocery store will always be there for you.

Ethnic Markets & Stores

Places like Hispanic Food Markets and Asian Food markets are amazing places to find uncommon meats, bones, organs and seafood that you would never see at your local grocery store. If you are someone that is not going to be able to source from online suppliers because of shipping costs then ethnic markets are going to be one of the biggest tools in your belt when it comes to variety and hard to find items like organs.

Online Sellers

Online sellers can be slightly more expensive because of shipping costs. It's also not something you can immediately get like food from the grocery store or hispanic and asian markets but they are without a doubt the best place to source varieties of food. What I tend to do is use online sellers to source foods that I can't find locally. This keeps a variety of food in my dogs' diets.

I personally order from www.rawfeedingmiami.com but there is no shortage of options when it comes to online sellers. I prefer Raw Feeding Miami not only because of their quality, but also because I have noticed a drastic difference in shipping costs with RFM compared to others, even with other suppliers that are the same distance from me. That being said, shipping rates change regularly and by location of delivery so be sure to do your homework and choose what works best for you.

Local Raw Pet Food Sources

If you are one of the people out there lucky enough to have a local manufacturer of raw pet food in their area then consider yourself lucky. I for example have Ford's Locker, a 70+ year family owned & operated business that processes game and produces a beef/elk/venison ground mix. They also ship if you want to look them up on Facebook. If you do have someone like this, do what you can do build a relationship with the owners. You never know what could come from it.

Butchers - Half & Half

In my personal opinion from observation over the years butchers are a half and half when it comes to consistent vs inconsistent sources. Depending on the butcher, the type of butcher they are, and the relationship you have with the butcher, the availability of cuts, scraps and other foods can vary. By all means, do not dismiss this option but be prepared to be told no by a few butchers before you are able to develop a good relationship with one who is willing to work with you.

This is not meant to be discouraging but even if you do establish a good relationship with a butcher there is just as much of a chance of them having scraps etc...available on a regular basis as there is for them to have these things on a sporadic basis.

Point being, unless you get really lucky you can't depend on the butcher being your one and only source for food.

Let's take a look at Inconsistent sources now.

What Is An Inconsistent Source?

Inconsistent sources are sources that can provide you with some truly excellent scores that, depending on your needs could set you up for months if you're lucky. That being said, they aren't sources that you can regularly rely on because there is no way to control their availability.

Some examples of inconsistent sources would include:
- Hunters
- Ad Sites
- Friends & Family
- Processing Plants

Hunters

Hunters are an absolutely amazing inconsistent source. Often times hunters are after prime cuts and/or heads to mount when they are hunting. This provides an opportunity for you to get all of the other meats and organs that the hunter has no plans to use. So if you know anyone that hunts, it's time to start making friends out of them. Always offer to come and take it, make it zero effort on their part. A single score from an elk or deer hunter can fill your freezer for a good long time. If you do score an elk, deer, or any other wild game that was shot with a firearm, do a thorough job of inspecting the food for any projectile fragments. In other words, make sure there aren't pellets or pieces of a bullet in the meat you are feeding. Typically these types of ammunition are made of lead and are highly toxic.

As a personal example, recently I received 45 lbs. of fresh, never frozen, all organic of course, Utah antelope. 100%, free of charge. All it took was one Facebook comment on a friend's post congratulating him on his kill and mentioning that I know 2 dogs that love scraps. The next day a cooler full of meat showed up at my house.

Ad Sites (Craigslist, etc...)

This is hit or miss but if you can construct a good post explaining that you feed a fresh, homemade diet to your dogs and that you are willing to take on unwanted meat from hunters or people cleaning out their freezers for whatever reason you can make some big scores.

Hunters do this a lot with freezer burnt meat from the last year's hunt and because freezer burnt meat is perfectly fine for your dog this is a real advantage for you. They may even raise and butcher livestock of some kind whether it be chickens, cows, or whatever and often have scraps to get rid of that they would part with for free or a very low price because it would get thrown away anyways.

One of my students of the Raw Feeding 101 online course used the ad template provided to them and scored more than 200 lbs of free meat in less than 48 hours.

Long story short, sometimes it works, sometimes it doesn't, but when it does work it can REALLY work.

Friends & Family

You'd be surprised at how often friends and family will contact you with scores of meat if you are simply open about the fact that you feed raw.

As another personal example, not too long ago I received 100 lbs of free beef from a friend of my wifes who's family had just butchered and processed a cow and had no need for the "non prime cuts" of meat. At an average of $3-$4 a pound for beef that's $300 - $400 worths of free meat.

Let that sink in for a minute...

Don't hide the fact that you feed raw. You could literally be letting money go down the drain.

Processing Plants

For a vast majority of raw feeders this can be the most inconsistent source but can be a huge score from time to time. If you have a processing plant near you whether it's for beef, pork, game, or whatever else, don't be afraid to reach out. Like the butcher though, don't expect to hear yes every time.

Ask to be put on a list of some kind to be contacted when scraps are available if at all possible.
If they happen to be a processing plant that also raises their livestock offer to come and retrieve fallen animals so long as they didn't die from disease.

As you can see there is no shortage of options for sourcing your food. When it comes to sourcing your food I would recommend that you do it in two steps.

1. Find Reliable Consistent Sources

Even if it is something as simple as grocery stores or ethnic markets, or both, secure those resources first.

Recently Florida was slammed in 2017 by the truly devastating string of hurricanes. While the residents obviously felt a much greater impact than we did, it did temporarily shut down one of our resources. Having other consistent sources allowed us to keep our boys fed with zero issue.

2. Dedicate Some Time To Finding Inconsistent Sources.

When it comes to inconsistent sources, putting in extra time is the name of the game.
Whether you are contacting butchers, putting up ads on Facebook or craigslist, building relationships with hunters, etc…the time you put in will make the difference.

So after you get your transition complete and have established reliable, consistent sources, start looking for those BIG inconsistent source scores.

Considerations For Small Dogs

One of the most annoying rumors that I hear on a regular basis online when it comes to raw feeding is that small dogs can't eat raw. This is of course absolutely ridiculous for plenty of reasons BUT there are some things that you want to consider if you are going to be feeding a small dog raw so let's go over those now.

Consideration #1 - Small Dog's Can't Eat Whole Bones

Gotcha! Sorry about the false title but that's exactly what it is, false. Lots of people say that small dogs simply can't chew bones and therefore HAVE to be fed ground raw food exclusively. That is not true, but this particular rumor IS based in some sliver of truth.

What I mean is that SOME small dogs DO have trouble with bones. Most of the time this is only with puppies of small breeds or small breeds in the beginning of their raw diet journey. The puppies usually grow out of this as they mature and the adult dogs get better with whole bones as time goes on but there are some things you can do to help this AND keep their raw diet going while they adjust

1. Feed Grinds

In the beginning some small breed dogs and puppies do best with grinds. It will allow them to adjust to the raw diet without also having to adjust to chewing whole bones. But that doesn't mean you should withhold whole bones entirely which brings me to #2.

2. Allow Them To Try Whole Bones.

This can be during meal time or can also be given as an extra special treat of some kind. Maybe one day a week you decide to feed your small breed dog or puppy a wing or neck from a chicken, turkey, duck, etc... and let them go at it long enough to figure things out or until they consume it.

Of course, make sure you are feeding an appropriately sized neck or wing. This again lets them get used to the whole process of chewing, allows them to develop their jaw, neck, and shoulder muscles as well as building dexterity with their arms and paws that allows them to hold the whole food while they chew.

Consideration #2 - Digital scales

When it comes to measuring out the different portions of your small dogs raw diet, it can be difficult because these amounts can be extremely small, ESPECIALLY when it comes to liver and other organs.

Having one of the "needle scales" where the needle moves along a graph as the weight on the scale increases simply isn't going to do the job. They're rarely sensitive enough to properly illustrate weights in those extremely small amounts.

To solve this problem you can use a digital scale. They are extremely cheap, are easy to use, and will allow you to get accurate weight measurements even with extremely small amounts of food.

Consideration #3 - Balancing Across A Week Instead Of Daily

Later in the book in the transition section I will address whether to balance your dog's meals on a daily basis or whether you should balance over time. In that section I am going to recommend doing it on a daily basis because it's easier to keep track of and it's easier to portion meals to freeze for later that way. AKA meal prep.

However, for small dogs it may be easier for some to balance over time. Which in it's simplest terms, or at least one definition, means to balance those daily amounts over a week.

For example, If you were supposed to feed 0.5 oz of bone per day but it was very hard to get that small of an amount into each meal, you may opt to feed 1 oz every other day, or even 1.5 oz every 3 days. The idea is to balance within a certain time frame instead of meal by meal.

Don't get me wrong, balancing day by day, meal by meal is still completely doable but many find it difficult to get the small amounts necessary into a single meal and prefer to feed it overtime like I just explained. Only you can make that call based on what foods are available to you and what you decide is best for you. You want to provide your dog with the best diet possible but you still need to do it in a way that is sustainable for you, as the feeder, effort wise.

So there you have it, a few really quick and really simple things to consider when feeding your small breed dog a raw diet. Whether it's a shih tzu, a chihuahua, beagle, toy poodle, or some other breed or mixed breed small dog, they are just as capable as any of the giant breeds out there of benefiting from a raw food diet.

Considerations For Senior Dogs

Do you have a senior dog you are wanting to transition to a raw diet? FANTASTIC! It's never too late to improve a dog's diet and by extension, their quality of life. That being said, there are some things that you as a senior dog owner should consider when making the switch and I want to address those things in this section

Let's get started!

Consideration #1 - Dental Factors

One of the biggest issues plaguing today's domestic canine is dental issues. Traditional dog food like kibble is a major factor in this. Considering the facts that your dog is not yet being fed raw and your dog is a senior, there is potential that dental issues have set in if they were not brought to the vet for regular cleanings.

So DOES your senior dog have any dental issues? You of course are the only one that can answer this question because I do not know your dog.

If your senior dog does not have any dental issues then GREAT! If there are some dental issues, you will need to proceed in a different manner.

If your senior dog's dental issues are purely cosmetic and they could just use a good cleaning then that's okay because raw feeding can go a long way when it comes to a good tooth cleaning. If your senior dog's dental issues are more severe and could prevent the chewing action necessary to eat whole foods, you may want to explore the option of feeding mostly to all ground raw foods, then of course provide chews whenever possible of some kind combined with veterinarian help to satisfy the tooth cleaning needs of your dog.

The last thing we want is for your dog to suffer on any level so if you believe with the help of your veterinarian that your dog may have difficulties handling the task of heavy chewing like chewing through the bones in whole food, ground raw may be the best option for YOUR dog.

Again, only you and your vet can truly gauge your dog's dental state so evaluate this carefully and make the best call from there.

Consideration #2 - Old Dogs & New Tricks

By the time we as human are adults we are long since established in our preferences of what it is that we do and do not like to eat. Your senior dog may not be so different.

It's not uncommon for senior dogs to have a sense of confusion when presented with raw because they have been fed kibble for years and years and may not understand that this new "stuff" is supposed to be dinner. Some senior dogs are simply picky snobs and don't want to change up their long-established routine and will turn their noses up when presented with raw. You may get lucky and your dog will immediately take to it.

If you aren't that lucky it's important to understand that you are not alone and that it is not an uncommon thing. Be patient, keep trying, and if worse comes to worse, start adding small amounts of raw to their commercial food (meat only) and when they start to show some interest, attempt the transition steps that you'll see later in the book again.

Consideration #3 - Slow Transitions

I always recommend slow transitions when it comes to making the switch which is why the transition process is set up in a 4+week/step block. That being said, some senior dogs will be exceptionally sensitive to the change.

Any dog has the potential to be sensitive to the change and need longer than others to transition but sometimes this can be more common in senior dogs. I mentioned earlier about senior dogs being sometimes picky and set in their ways, well sometimes their bodies are the same way.

It may take longer at the age they are at now to transition than it would have taken them say 5 years ago.

Just like the mentally picky eater, provide the body with the same courtesy. Be patient, take your time if you have to, and move through the transition steps when the body tells you it's ready to move on to the next step.

I'll go over that in greater detail in the transition portion of the book.

To wrap up I want to simply say this. Our senior dogs are great companions. For many of us they have been with us for years and years but if you adopted a senior dog that may not be the case. Either way they are amazing little (or maybe not so little) creatures in their golden years and are just as capable of making the transition to a raw diet. They just may need a special touch to do so.

Be patient, understand the possible challenges a senior dog may face, and don't give up.

Sodium & What You Need To Know

In this section I want to cover something that is easy to overlook but is super important. It's also something that a lot of new raw feeders don't find out about until they are well into their raw feeding journey. That easy to overlook and super important thing is the sodium content in your dog's diet.

Let's get started!

According to a work published by the National Academy Of Sciences, a dog's diet should consist of no more than 100mg -

200mg of sodium a day. This provides the body with the necessary amount of sodium but is not enough to cause the issues associated with elevated amounts of sodium. Too much sodium in a dogs diet can cause a lot of problems that ranges from simple nausea to weakness, lack of energy, vomiting, and in extreme cases vet visits.

So With This In Mind How Do You Know How Much To Feed?

Well with the combined information from the national academy of sciences and the raw feeding community as we know it today, we have an easy to follow guideline that can be used to keep our dogs safe.

This guideline is not providing foods that contain more than approx. 100mg of sodium per 4 oz. Serving. That is the "how much". It doesn't sound like a lot but you may be surprised.

In today's chicken industry, a lot of suppliers "plump" their birds with a solution that is high in sodium to make the birds both weight more and appear larger. It's not uncommon in today's commercially available chicken to get upwards of 500mg of sodium per 4 oz. Serving.

So How Do You Control This 100mg Per 4 oz Serving?

There are two really good ways to do this.

First, you can buy your raw food from a provider that does not add any solutions, or sodium, or anything else to their food. Lots of online suppliers fit this bill. Online providers like Raw Feeding Miami and Hare-today. If for some reason you are unable to source your raw food from places like this, you have a second option.

When purchasing raw food from somewhere other than a source that does not add solutions or sodium to their food it's important to read the label. Most packaging for raw foods like chicken as an example, have nutritional information. Two of these pieces of information are the sodium amount and serving size which you can use to make sure you are close to the recommended 100mg per 4 oz serving or below.

For example, if you look at the package of raw food and it says a serving is 16 oz and contains 400mg of sodium per 16 oz serving, you know it's a safe food to feed.

We know this because simple math tells us that 4 oz. Is ¼ of the foods total serving size and ¼ of the total sodium content is 100mg so you are good to go.

I did not keep sodium in mind when I first started and I really wish I had. I was lucky enough to not experience any significant issues from it but that's just the thing, I got lucky.

Don't be me.

It may seem like a pain in the butt but with a little attention to where you source your food from and/or a little label reading you can avoid all of the problems associated with providing too much sodium in your dog's diet.

Chapter 4

Feeding Raw Foods & What You Need To Know

Chapter Explanation

In this section I want to cover a few quick things about some of the foods that you may or may not end up feeding your dog. I want to explain exactly what the food is, and some best practices when it comes to feeding that food.

So let's get to the first section.

Feeding Muscle Meat - The 80%

Here we are going to talk about muscle meat or "The 80%" and some things you need to know about feeding it.

What Is The 80% or Muscle Meat?

Like we discussed in the "Secret Formula" section. Muscle meat is going to take up the largest portion of your dog's diet. Muscle meat is exactly what it sounds like, muscle meats from the animals that you will be feeding. There are a few exceptions to this depending on how you think about it like green tripe but for the most part this is the case. There are also a few things that are technically organs like heart and giblets that are fed as meat.

I know that seems confusing but that's pretty much where the confusion ends. Muscle meat is muscle tissue.

What dogs can eat it?

All dogs on a raw diet should be receiving a large amount of muscle meat. There is virtually no exception to this rule. There are some dogs with severe allergies to a range of protein/meat sources so some dogs may be limited to the variety of proteins that they can have. Canines NEED large amounts of protein from muscle meat in order to thrive. Too much protein can of course be harmful but as long as you follow the secret formula you should be okay.

Just to clarify, when we say "proteins" in the raw feeding world we are talking about the muscle meat from a specific animal. I.E. beef is one protein and chicken is another. Okay, moving on.

What dogs should stay away from it?

Like I just mentioned, dogs on a raw diet WILL need large amounts of muscle meat.
The only real exception to this rule is going to be dogs that have allergies to certain proteins that I just went over.

How to use/feed it?

There are several ways to feed the 80% portion of the diet. Some people feed it whole, some people feed it ground, and some people chop it into varying sizes. It all depends on what you have chosen to do with your method of feeding and what your dog will and will not accept.

For example, I know a lot of people with dogs that do not like eating whole so their owners are forced to cut the food into smaller pieces in order for their dogs to eat it.

It's also extremely important to note that a wide variety of muscle meat should be fed. Different proteins contain different levels of fats, amino acids, minerals, and so on. Most shoot for at least 3-4 different proteins which is easier to do than you would think, but the more proteins you can rotate in your dog's diet the better. This difference in amino acids is particularly important when comparing red meat to white meat. Ideally, you want to shoot for around 50% red meat and 50% white meat. If you feed one more than the other, try to feed more red meat than white meat. Don't just feed chicken meat, but feed chicken, beef, duck, turkey, pork and so on. Whatever you do, don't feed a diet comprised of a single protein unless you have one of the rare dogs that can only handle one protein for medical reasons. This circumstance should be diagnosed by a licensed veterinarian, preferably a holistic one.

So there you have it, the 80% is extremely straightforward and simple. Feed approximately 80% muscle meat and adjust when necessary according to your dog's needs. You might have to cut it into pieces or grind it but whatever you do, get it into the diet. It's crucial.

Feeding Bone - The 10%

In this section we are going to talk about bone or "The 10%" and some things you need to know about feeding it.

Bones are one of the scariest things for new feeders. Like we talked about in the overcoming mental barriers section people have been programmed into thinking that bones are dangerous and should never ever be fed to dogs. While you now know this to be true with cooked bones, it certainly isn't with raw bones.

What dogs can eat it?

ALL dogs on a raw diet should have bone in their diet. Raw bones are high in both calcium and phosphorus which are key in the development and support of the immune system, bone growth, tooth growth and a plethora of other things.

This is ESPECIALLY true when it comes to growing puppies.

Just like the 80% muscle meat, the 10% bone content MUST be in the diet. There are certain situations where bones need to be ground or eggshells are provided for additional calcium. You should note that eggshells do not provide all the same things that bones do so they are not a suitable permanent replacement for bones.

What bones should dogs stay away from?

When it comes to feeding raw bones the vast majority of bones are fine to eat, but I highly recommend you stay away from the weight bearing bones of large animals.

When I say a weight bearing bones I mean anything that is responsible for supporting the weight of the animal. But again this is specific to large animals. The weight bearing bones of large animals are far too dense to be fed on a regular basis without causing some kind of dental wear or even cracked / broken teeth.

For example, the legs of a chicken, while technically being weight bearing bones, are completely fine to feed because the animal is small and the bones are not extremely dense. The bones in the leg of a cow, elk, or deer fall into the class of weight bearing bones that should not be fed. They are far too dense and tend to cause the wear and broken teeth I just discussed.

Some people do still offer these larger, more dense bones and will tell you that feeding large bones like this is fine but I would highly suggest you not follow in their steps.

It's all fun and games until someone shatters a molar or canine tooth.

How to use/feed it?

Much like the 80% muscle meat there are several ways to feed bone. The most obvious is whole. This would include raw meaty bones like chicken quarters, the necks from birds like duck, turkey, and chicken, pork ribs, bird frames, heads for those that are ready for that, and so on.

Another option that is often chosen by those with dogs that have dental issues or who are simply too afraid to give their dogs whole bones is to feed ground food that includes ground bone. These are called grinds more often than not.

The other way that people feed bone is getting ground bone and adding to food themselves. I
find this method to be tiresome and unnecessary so unless you simply cannot get past feeding whole bones and for some reason don't want to feed grinds, just don't bother.

Alright, that's bones. I know that for several of you the "cut and dry" nature of this section may be a little underwhelming but it's on purpose. While I completely understand the hesitation and concern that is caused by the clever marketing I discussed earlier in the book, the mental aspect of feeding bones truly is the most complicated part about it. Remember, dogs are canines. To put it bluntly, they are biomechanical machines engineered by mother nature herself to hunt, kill, and eat other animals...including their bones.

Follow the advice above and trust mother nature.

We'll talk more about figuring out how much to feed later with the bone calculator provided with this book.

Feeding Liver & Non-liver Organs - The 5% & 5%

In this section we are going to talk about liver and non-liver organs or "The 5%" and "The OTHER 5%" and some things you need to know about feeding it.

While the "what liver is" is pretty self explanatory, what "non-liver organ" is can be a little more confusing. Non-liver organ is any secreting organ within the animals we feed that is not liver.

Again, there are some organs that we feed as muscle meat like the heart and gizzards.
The list of non-liver, secreting organs you will be feeding as part of "the OTHER 5%" include organs like the spleen, pancreas, kidneys, brain, and reproductive organs like ovaries and testicles.

Both liver and non-liver organs are extremely important in the dog's diet and are considered the most vitamin, mineral, and overall nutrient dense parts of the diet. These organs provide nutritional value that simply can't be found in the muscle meat or bones of the animal.

This is one of the reasons organs were so prized among native humans across the world. Unrelated? Yes, but still interesting and it makes a point.

It's also important to feed a variety of both liver and non-liver organs just like I discussed in regards to proteins. By variety I mean, not just feeding chicken liver but rotating chicken liver, beef liver, turkey liver, etc...Feeding liver from a wide variety of animals. The same goes for non-liver organs.

Variety, variety, variety. Have I mentioned variety is important?

Choosing not to feed liver and non-liver organs is choosing to not feed a balanced diet, in which case staying on kibble would be a better idea.

You're of course not going to do that so make sure to keep the liver and non-liver organs in the diet.

How to use/feed it?

Feeding organs can sometimes be extremely difficult. Not in the actual feeding but getting your dog to eat it. It's not so weird if you think about it. Most organs, are gelatinous, slimy, have strong tastes, and can smell a little weird. Sometimes I think our dogs agree with us on this one.

You can combat this in 3 ways.

1. Feed it frozen or partially frozen.

Organs defrost very quickly so don't pull them out of the freezer hours before feeding time.
When you feed frozen organs, it mellows out the flavor and changes the consistency making it less slimy which can help you trick that picky eater.

2. Blend it and feed as a liquid.

I had to use this method to get my dogs to eat organs. Simply take your liver and non-liver organs and put them in a food processor or blender depending on the quantity you want to make. Start with a small amount at first to see if your dog will eat it. Then mix in an egg and a spoonful of coconut oil and blend it all together into a liquid.

The exact measurements are not necessarily important on this one, all you are trying to do is mask the flavor of the organs a bit and again change the texture. You can then feed as a liquid or freeze it. Again, the goal here is to trick the picky eater.

3. Grind it with other foods.

If you are lucky enough to have a grinder or even a heavy duty food processor then you will be able to grind your organs up with other food items like muscle meat and possibly fruits/veggies. By doing this you are again masking the taste and changing the texture in hopes of tricking your lil' picky eater.

The bottomline is that if your dog is going to refuse a particular food during their raw feeding journey it is probably going to be liver or non-liver organs. If you follow these 3 tricks you should be able to get past that and be able to feed whole organs without any extra prep.

Again, organs are EXTREMELY important. Under no circumstance should you omit these from the diet unless you are doing so under the advisement of a raw educated veterinarian.

The last thing I want to mention in regards to organs before we move on is that they often cause loose stools/runs for dogs that are new to the raw diet. We will go over this more in chapter 7, the transition chapter but it is extremely common and I felt it was necessary to at least mention it in this section.

Feeding Chicken & What You Need To Know

In this section we are going to talk about chicken and some things you need to know about feeding it.

Chicken is the highest produced animal in the world and almost all of us are eating it, our dogs included. Chicken is the most commonly recommended protein to start with because it's a white meat protein, the bones are soft, it's inexpensive, and it's readily available.

There is a downside though.

Like I mentioned, chicken is the most commonly produced animal in the world, because of this they also receive the most medicine, the most antibiotics, and so on. For some dogs this causes issues, their bodies simply don't react well to it.

Chicken is also one of the most common protein intolerances I see in dogs.

While I believe a lot of these allergic dogs may actually be reacting to the drugs or food the chickens are fed and not the chicken itself, the point remains that chicken can't be fed to those dogs.

That sounds like a whole lot of negatives but don't discount chicken just yet. Remember, it's a white meat protein which is the type of meat you will be starting with, it has extremely soft bones so they're ideal for nervous and newbie raw feeders, is extremely inexpensive, and can be found at almost every grocery store around the world.

Unless you already know your dog has issues with chicken or you simply can't get ahold of it I recommend starting your raw feeding journey with chicken.
If problems arise then move onto another white meat like turkey or rabbit.

Feeding Eggs & What You Need To Know

In this section we are going to talk about eggs and some things you need to know about feeding them.

Eggs are an AMAZING food to add to your dog's raw diet. They are jam packed full of protein, 6+ grams of protein per egg to be exact, contains 13 essential vitamins and minerals, and can even reduce hunger in dogs on a diet. They contain a good source of fatty acids, vitamin A, vitamin b12, iron, and more. They have been referred to as "nature's multivitamin".

As amazing as eggs are, you will want to be cautious if you are feeding the shells from high production, commercial companies. The shells are often washed and exposed to chemicals which in high enough concentrations over time can be hurtful. Buy organic whenever possible or even better find them from a local seller or raise chickens yourself.

In the past a lot of people have made a big deal out of biotin deficiency caused by feeding eggs which couldn't be more wrong...well mostly.

The key is to feed the WHOLE EGG. Not just the whites, but the whole egg.

While it is true that the egg whites can cause a biotin deficiency if fed in large amounts, feeding the yolk which is very high in biotin essentially balances out this whole "egg equation". It's also important to note that while biotin plays other roles in the body, one of the most physically apparent benefits is the support of a healthy coat. If you see a dog with a lack luster coat it's possible they are experiencing a biotin deficiency.

Another common misconception about feeding eggs is the fear of salmonella. Just as your dog will be safe when they eat a high quality source of chicken, your dog will be perfectly fine with feeding FRESH raw eggs so long as you have a healthy dog with a properly functioning immune system.

Dogs were designed by nature to ingest and eliminate small amounts of harmful bacteria like salmonella so as long as your dog is healthy and you are providing, again, FRESH eggs then all will be well. If you can't get fresh eggs then simply avoid feeding the shell.

How often to feed it?

Some people will feed eggs as often as every day for it's benefits with the coat and more, some people don't feed them at all. I would start off with one egg or two a week and move on to a few a week (3-4) depending on your dog's size and go from there. There isn't a perfect answer.

Feeding Fish & What You Need To Know

In this section we are going to talk about fish and some things you need to know about feeding it.

Soooo fish, there's a lot that's been said over the last several years about feeding raw fish so here is what you need to know.

Why would we want to feed fish?

Well, fish contains omega 3 fatty acids which are essential to the health of canines. We can supplement with things like fish oil, krill oil, or phytoplankton but some people prefer to get the omega 3s from whole foods. Fish is also a great source of vitamin D which dogs cannot manufacture on their own from sunlight like some other animals do.

What's the scare all about?

More and more of the waters on our planet are contaminated with mercury, pesticides, chemicals, and toxic metals. These nasty things in one way or another ends up in the bodies of the fish that we would like to be feeding to our dogs. The larger the fish and the longer they live the more contaminated they can be.

Because of this, it's important that if you choose to feed fish you keep a few things in mind.

Fish With Short Lifespans

Go for fish that do not have long lifespans and are known to have lower levels of mercury. A great source for this is sardines. You can find them in the can at most grocery stores. Other great options include anchovies, herring, mackerel, smelt, trout, and salmon. Smelt is our preferred choice because they are inexpensive and easy to find.

Pay Close Attention To Sourcing

It used to be easy to simply say that including wild salmon in your dog's diet as part of the rotation was good enough. As our waters become more and more contaminated, even this comes into question. So if you choose to feed salmon make sure you are doing your research and finding the best source possible. This is going to be heavily dependent on where that salmon comes from so again do your research.

Freeze

Some people say to kill parasites like worms that could be present in raw fish, it's necessary to freeze the fish for a week. Some say as little as 24 hours is sufficient but personally I don't feel like that's enough. Especially if you have an underperforming freezer.

I recommend freezing for a few weeks before feeding any raw fish, especially if you caught it yourself. There is an exception to this rule when it comes to feeding fish from sources that freeze it beforehand like rawfeedingmiami.com.

Additionally if one of your sources of fish is the local river, stream, or lake, it's important to completely gut the fish and check the body, including the head for hooks.

You never know when the last time that fish got caught and released. The last thing you want is to end up at the vet because your dog swallowed a fish hook.

How often should you feed it?

A do not feel that fish should ever be the sole protein in a dogs diet or even a significant portion of the diet. Like everything else, I think it should be a part of the rotation.

If you choose to use supplementation like fish oil or the other options I discussed, make sure to read the instructions carefully as they can vary in recommended amounts.
The general recommended amount is approximately 10mg per 10 lbs of body weight.

It's also important to note that when it comes to supplementing with fish oil that you choose a product that is 3rd party tested for quality and authenticity in their claims.

If you choose to feed whole fish pay very close attention to sourcing, where the fish was sourced from, what type of fish it is, and so on like we've already discussed. Feed approx. 1 oz per 30-35 lbs of bodyweight when fed.

If you feed one then it's not necessary to feed the other. In other words if you are going to supplement with fish oil 4 days a week, and feed whole fish 3 days a week, you don't need feed them on the same day.

So that's fish. It's a lot to consider.

Personally my wife and I have chosen to go with a high quality, 3rd party tested fish oil for our dog Wolken, who can't eat fish. Partly for convenience, but mostly because for one reason or another, all types of fish makes him vomit.

For our dog Horus we go with a combination of locally sourced smelt and the same fish oil Wolken has.

Whatever you decide to do, think it through, do your research, and make the best choice possible.

Feeding Fruits & Vegetables & What You Need To Know

In this section we are going to talk about fruits & vegetables and some things you need to know about feeding it.

Should dogs be eating fruits & vegetables?

You will not find a more highly debated topic when it comes to raw feeding.

The opinions of most people on one side or the argument or the other are well, extreme. Some think that there is no way a dog should be without fruits and vegetables while others believe that there is no place in the raw diet for fruits and vegetables.

Typically these two groups are sectioned into B.A.R.F. feeders believing in fruits and vegetables on one side and the prey model / whole prey feeders believing the opposite on the other side.

Luckily, there is a growing number of people within a third group that simply believes in raw feeding and believes that it is a personal choice to feed them or not to feed them.

When I recorded my Raw Feeding 101 online video course I was still on the fence about vegetables. I didn't necessarily believe they were harmful, but I definitely didn't feel like they were highly beneficial.

I've since changed my tune.

I always tell my course students, my Facebook group members, my 1 on 1 coaching students and social media followers to NOT get stuck in their ways with any one particular part of raw feeding.

For years I did exactly that.

More and more information has been coming out about the benefits of vegetables and the impact they could have (especially when fermented) on the dog's microbiome, immune system, and overall health.

I've been feeding raw for a little less than 9 years, and as I type this chapter I am currently in the process of adding fermented vegetables to my dogs' diets. Why you ask? Good question. Because the amount of evidence to support the benefits has become simply too much for me to ignore.

My goal in feeding my dogs a raw diet isn't to adhere to any one particular model of raw feeding, it's to keep my dogs as healthy as possible for as long as possible so they LIVE as long as possible. I now believe that fermented vegetables are going to help me in that goal.

Now I'm not saying that you need to do the same, rather I encourage you dive as deep as possible into the veggie pool and make the decision for yourself. I also hope that you consider the fact that a 9-year raw feeder like myself is changing my tune when it comes to feeding vegetables. I'm not trying to sway your opinion, I'm just saying that at this point my raw feeding journey, it takes a lot of convincing and good information for me to make major changes in my dogs' diets.

What dogs should stay away from it?

There are some dogs out there that seem to have constant battles with yeast whether this yeast is found in their paws, ears, and so on. If you are an owner of one of these dogs it may be in your best interest to really think about whether or not you are going to feed vegetables.

The reason for this is that there are lots of vegetables out there that have high amount of starch and starch can essentially feed your dog's yeast problems. So if you are going to feed vegetables and have one of these dogs do your research and make sure you are only feeding low glycemic or low starch vegetables like kale, spinach, and asparagus.

The bottom line is that vegetables and fruits are a highly debated topic in the raw feeding world with some people thinking they are highly beneficial, and others think they have no place in a dog's diet.

The transition portion of the book will get you through your first 4 weeks/steps and will be a prey model based transition. During this 4-week transition period I encourage you to continue your research and come to your own conclusion of whether or not you will feed fruits and vegetables.

Feeding Green Tripe & What You Need To Know

In this section we are going to talk about green tripe and some things you need to know about feeding it.

So what exactly IS green tripe?

Green tripe is the stomach of ruminating animals like beef, goats, and sheep. Green tripe is a great source of natural enzymes, protein, probiotics, healthy fats, is jam packed full of vitamins and nutrients, and has a healthy calcium to phosphorus ratio.

Another "benefit" is that it stinks like nothing you've smelled before. If you have ever encountered a smell as...strong...as green tripe, you do not have my envy. The reason I say this is a benefit is because that strong odor that makes you want to put on a hazmat suit is extremely enticing to your dog.
Because of this it is great if you have a picky eater that either won't eat certain foods, or hates the taste of supplements like fish oil.

We use green tripe for all the reasons above including the stench. Although truthfully after handling it a few times you never notice. If you can change a diaper, you can feed green tripe. The stench helps us make a beautiful little concoction of green tripe, topped with fish oil and finally drenched in a ph supplement.

The dogs love it so much that they've been known to lap that whole mixture up first before touching any of the other food in that day's meal.

How is it fed?

Green tripe often comes in 3 main forms. Ground, chunked, and whole.
I find it SOOOO much easier to buy and feed ground, that way I can be much more specific with the amounts I'm feeding.

On top of that, there are no additional steps like cutting up the whole green tripe. It also allows me to create the concoction I described. Like anything else, you should introduce it slowly to give your dog time to adjust to the new food. I recommend adding it into the diet after the initial transition as part of the 80% muscle meat category.

The exact amount of the 80% that you feed as green tripe is up to you but I prefer to use it as a daily natural "supplement" because of all of it's probiotic, enzyme, and vitamin/mineral properties. To achieve this "supplemental" type feeding I will generally make 10-15% of the 80% muscle meat.

I will caution you on feeding too much however.

While green tripe is extremely nutrient dense, it is a lower calorie food. Feeding too much may cause unintentional weight loss. That being said, if weight loss is something you are looking for, temporarily increasing the amount of green tripe may help your dog hit those weight loss goals.

So all in all green tripe is well, amazing. Between the natural enzymes, vitamins and minerals, calcium phosphorus balance, high protein content and on and on it's easy to see why this food is seen as a "Canine super food".

The only thing that stinks about green tripe is well...it stinks.

Feeding Grinds & Premades & What You Need To Know

In this section we are going to talk about premades & grinds and some things you need to know about feeding it.

What are grinds and premades?

Grinds and premades do differ from each other slightly but they are essentially premade & ground raw food. Let's address them each specifically so you know what the differences between the two are.

Grinds

Grinds are multiple parts of an animal ground together. For example, a duck grind would most likely include the muscle meat, bones, organs and more all ground together to make a "grind". Basically, taking all of the ingredients of a prey model diet and grinding them together.
Grinds are typically sold in chubs and pouch type packages and a wide range of proteins are available in grinds from duck to turkey, chicken, fish and more.

Premades

Premades are similar in the fact that they are multiple ingredients ground together but often times premades are not exclusively prey model type ingredients.

For example a premade may contain chicken meat and chicken bones, the liver and possibly another organ from the chicken, as well as fruits and/or veggies. Premades come in a variety of forms like patties, nuggets, and chubs and are also available in a wide range of proteins.

In my opinion the most important thing to remember when it comes to feeding grinds or premades is that they may not be balanced when it comes to the 80/10/5/5 formula which means you'll have to balance it on your own.

For example, there are lots of premades out there that only include liver and do not include any non-liver organs. It's my opinion that this should be corrected by you adding a non-liver organ to their meals. The problem with this is that there is not always easily available information when it comes to the exact or even approximate amounts and ratios of what is in these premade raw foods.

This means you are going to have to do a little detective work and possibly contact the company yourself. When you find out what is in it, all you have to do is compare it to the 80/10/5/5 formula and fill in the blanks just like the example I just shared about the the premade that did not contain a non-liver organ.

We identified what was missing and added it ourselves.

Something to consider when it comes to grinds and premades is that you will essentially be using it as a cold turkey transition method. In essence you are doing a balanced from the start method depending on how complete the grind or premade is. To put it simply, you have no choice but to do a "balanced from the start" approach because all the different food items are already mixed together.

I already mentioned the difference between slow transitions and balanced from the start transitions earlier in the book so make sure you keep the things I talked about in mind if you are going to use grinds and/or premades as a transition method.

Cost

The last thing we need to discuss about grinds and premades, especially premades, is the cost.

Almost without exception (and I say almost just to be safe but I can't think of any brands of premade that this doesn't apply for) premades are significantly more expensive than DIY raw. DIY raw meaning you are putting together the ingredients of the diet yourself.

Just like everything else, you are paying for convenience. Someone has already done the majority if not all of the work FOR YOU. I know a lot of people that do DIY raw who would gladly transition to premades and balance where necessary if it was more cost effective. Myself included.

In conclusion, there are a few things to keep in mind when it comes to feeding grinds and premades. They can be excellent raw food sources especially if the idea of putting everything together yourself is intimidating. You need to keep in mind that they come with some problems like balancing grinds and premades if it ends up being necessary. Most importantly, at least for those of us that don't have deep pockets, the cost of grinds and premades compared to putting together your own DIY raw yourself is significant.

Feeding Pork & What You Need To Know

In this section we are going to talk about pork and some things you need to know about feeding it.

Whether to feed pork or not is another widely debated topic in the raw feeding world. This is mainly due to a fear of the dogs contracting the trichinella disease. Trichinella used to be a huge concern when it came to U.S. pork raised for human consumption. According to the CDC between 1975 and 1981 there were nearly 800 reported cases of trichinella in the U.S. population that was largely caused by pork products.

This problem however has been long since and largely dealt with. According again to the CDC between 2008 and 2010 there were less than 50 reported cases of trichinella and approximately 10% of that was caused by pork based products.

This is one of the reasons why it upsets me when I see people in online raw feeding forums like Facebook, scaring new or prospective raw feeders by saying that their dogs will get sick from trichinella if they feed pork.

Now we do need to be fair and take into account that the CDCs numbers were reported cases of humans contracting the disease from varying levels of cooked food. That being said, the numbers still show an absolutely massive decline in the prevalence of trichinella. I for one have no problem with feeding pork that was raised for human consumption and I do. I feed pork on a weekly basis and have for years and years and I have never once had a problem.

But is it different with wild pigs? Yes.

There is a big difference when it comes to pigs raised for human consumption in controlled and regulated environments and wild hogs.

The risk of trichinella in wild pigs along with other diseases like pseudorabies is much higher and I cannot in good conscience recommend that you feed it. That being said, there are some raw feeding suppliers online that will sell it and a large number of people do feed it without issue. So if you want to go down that road I recommend doing a large amount of research into that company, their sourcing, and their quality control.

Again though, I would never recommend or support the idea of hunting wild hogs and feeding it to your dogs.

So what is the bottom line here? The bottom line here is that while trichinella was once a great issue here in the U.S. that is no longer the case and we have science from reputable sources like the CDC to show us this.

If you are feeding pork raised for human consumption in regulated environments then you will almost certainly not run into problems. However, if you go out and hunt a wild boar and feed this to your dog, well cross your fingers and hope you are one of the lucky ones.

Feeding Wild Caught Foods & What You Need To Know

In this section we are going to talk about wild caught meats and some things you need to know about feeding it.

So what qualifies as wild caught food?

Well that's simple. Did you get it from the grocery store or other local market? Did you get it from an online supplier? Or did you get it yourself via hunting, fishing, trapping, road kill, etc..?
If you said no to every question but the last one then you are most likely feeding wild caught food. This could be a deer or elk that you hunted. This could include animals like rabbits and squirrels that you caught in a live trap because they were a nuisance on your property. This could also include that trout that you and your buddy or family member caught this morning or last weekend. It may have even been that deer that was hit by a truck a block away from your house.

If it was alive in the wild before it was in your possession it counts as wild caught food.

Freezing

When it comes to feeding wild caught food, I always recommend freezing it for at least a few weeks. (3-4 or more if you want to get exact.) This is to kill a large number of freezing temperature sensitive parasites that could be passed on to your animal. It's important to note that freezing will not kill everything on the planet. That being said, if the animal you are going to feed was overall a healthy animal then you should be good to feed that animal after a few weeks of freezing.

Organs

Some whole prey feeders would disagree with me but it is my personal opinion that you should closely inspect ALL organs from a wild caught animal before feeding it. This can generally be accomplished by cutting into the organ. A heart or liver would be an excellent example.

What you are looking for is any sign of disease, worms, or other parasites. These are easily identifiable with a few quick google searches. **IMPORTANT NOTE* If you find an organ infested with a parasite or potential disease like flukes in the liver, you should not feed it even after freezing it. These infestations are typically highly concentrated if the infestation is present on any level so it just isn't worth the risk in my opinion.

Rabbits & Waterfowl

Some species of rabbit and waterfowl can be infested by a worm that lives in the muscle tissue of these animals and often times appears as small grains of rice in that muscle tissue.

With this in mind (again whole prey feeders may disagree) it is important to skin wild rabbit and waterfowl before feeding to confirm this worm isn't present.

If you find these rice like worms in that rabbit or waterfowl you shot you should get rid of it in my opinion.

It's again just not worth the risk in my humble opinion.

Fish

Recreational fishing is popular all over the world from Japan to the U.S. and more. As a raw feeder it would be easy to make the connection between fishing and your dog eating raw to meaning free food. You're right, it can be an amazing source of free meat for your dog. Like everything else we've talked about though it comes with unique risks and should be frozen for several weeks before feeding.

On top of freezing, it is important to completely gut fish and closely inspect the head and gills of fish. The reason for this is fish hooks and fishing line. The last thing you want to do is go to the vet because your dog swallowed a fish hook or fishing line without you or your dog knowing it.

Just because you took your hook out of the fish after you caught it does not mean another fisherman didn't catch that fish earlier and didn't do the same before releasing it.

Better safe than sorry because that sorry could cause your dog permanent damage, at the worst it could take their life, and at the best it will be a heavy burden on your bank account.

The bottomline when it comes to feeding wild caught food can be summed up in a few words, freeze & inspect.

If you freeze before feeding and inspect the food then you will be good to go more often than not.

Wild caught food can be extremely cost effective, an awesome addition to your diet when it comes to variety, and can even be fun if you're spending a quiet Sunday hunting or fishing to bring home food for the furry family members and human family members alike.

Chapter 5

Raw Food Meal Prepping

What Is Meal Prepping & Why Should You Bother?

In this section I want to talk about raw feeding meal prep. What it means and what are some of the benefits. You know, what the heck is it and why should you bother. Let's get to it.

Raw feeding meal prep, what is it?

Well it's exactly what it sounds like. Meal prep is the preparation of meals ahead of time for future use. This could be a week's worth, 2 weeks worth, a month's worth, it's all dependent on your supply of ingredients and your storage space.

So why should you bother? What ARE the benefits of doing meal prep or preparing meals ahead of time for your dog or dogs?

Benefit # 1 - It makes daily feeding easier.

When all you have to do is pull food out of the freezer and defrost that food it makes the idea of feeding raw a lot more manageable.

Benefit #2 - It makes daily feeding take less time.

In today's world time is a huge concern. We're constantly zipping from one project to another, sometimes juggling two or more at once. So when prospective raw feeders start thinking about the time it will take to feed raw compared to the time it takes to feed kibble that acts as an immediate turn off.

Again, when all you have to do is pull food out of the freezer to defrost, it drastically cuts down on the amount of time it will take on a daily basis to feed raw.

Benefit #3 - If you buy in bulk and prep all of it at once it can help you save money.

Like anything else in this world raw food can be significantly cheaper if you buy it in bulk.
A lot of online suppliers and even more so, co-ops provide discounted per pound costs if you are buying your food in bulk. This means you can spend less money and get more food if you are willing to get it all at once and do a round of meal preps

This of course will require you to have storage space but we'll talk about that more later.

Benefit #4 - It makes balancing meals easier for beginners.

For some people balancing over time is easier. I am not one of those people. I know that for me and I'm sure many others, I would end up forgetting things which would result in inconsistent balancing of my dogs diet and on top of that it's just one more thing to remember and manage throughout my week. Remember what i said about us all being so busy? I don't know about you but I don't need another thing to keep track of.

That's why balancing daily works out so well for me. When you prepare meals ahead of time you can balance each meal individually in rapid succession. It's a literal one and done when it comes to time and effort. You spend a couple of hours on a single day balancing a large number of meals and you're good to go for potentially weeks at a time.

This way I know that no matter how frizzle fried my brain gets throughout the week while I try and manage a business, a social media presence, a YouTube channel, spending time with my wife and dogs, and life in general, I won't end up forgetting something which would result in an imbalance or at least inconsistency in my dogs' diets.

Benefit #5 - Meal prepping works for all raw feeding types and models.

Fruits and veggies or no fruits and veggies? Fish or omega 3 oils? Whole bones or ground bones? There are lots of inconsistencies in raw feeding with all the different people defending their particular type of raw feeding and the way they do things. Meal prep however is one thing that everyone has in common.

It doesn't matter if you feed prey model, whole prey, BARF, grinds, premades, or a hybrid diet of some kind, meal prepping is something that everyone can do. The only thing that changes is what you're putting into the containers that will end up in the freezer.

Importance Of A Meal Prepping System

In this section I want to talk about having a system in place when it comes to your meal prepping. No, I don't mean some type of software on your computer or app on your phone but a PLAN. Having a system in place for your raw feeding meal preps is one of the most important things you can do. Let's talk about why for a minute.

Having a system in place or having a plan is one of the best favors you can do for yourself when it comes to meal prepping and by extension raw feeding in general. Now I know that this is already sounding like "Great, there's another thing I have to do." But I promise, it's no big deal at all. Just a simple system that lets you know what you are doing when and where. Let's go over what a good system will need and I think you'll be pleasantly surprised at just how easy it is to put together a new system that works well for you.

First, you'll need to decide where you are going to do your meal prep. Some people are super lucky and have dedicated areas in their homes that their friends, spouse, or they themselves build in a garage, or basement where they do their meal preps. While it doesn't necessarily sound appealing to meal prep out in your garage for some people, it does come with advantages like not having to worry about messes in your home as much.

Personally, I do all the meal prepping for the dogs in our household and I do it in our kitchen.
The kitchen is the best option if you are going to do it in your home for most people because pretty much EVERYONE has some form of hard surface as flooring in the kitchen. Tile, vinyl, sealed wood floors, linoleum, etc… The important thing that all these surfaces have in common is that they are mostly flat, easy to clean, and most importantly, easy to sanitize.

Second, you are going to need to decide where everything is going to go. Take 5 quick minutes and really think this one through. Try and keep the things you are going to use the most, like food the closest to you and the things you are only going to use a handful of times farther away like your food containers that are going to end up in the freezer.

Really think this one through. It will be the difference between you being relaxed and standing still for the majority of your meal prepping and running around constantly. Where is your main prep area going to be, where you do the bulk of your work like cutting, weighing, etc…? Where are you going to keep your food? (This should be very close to your main prep area.) Where are your containers going to go? Do you have quick access to a sink where you can drain bags of sealed food like you'll receive if you get food from an online supplier like rawfeedingmiami.com?

I know this list doesn't make things SEEM like a simple system but really, once you think it through for 5 minutes it's no biggie. What it really boils down to is "What are you going to need?" This would include food, equipment, a sink, and where are you going to put everything including you in your main prep area.

For example, my system is as follows. My defrosted bulk foods go on the kitchen table that is easily cleaned and sanitized like everything else I'm about to list. The foods that I've taken in smaller amounts for immediate use goes in 4 pans on top of the stove. One for organs, one for meaty bone content, one for muscle meat, and one for parts of the 80% that I'll be using smaller amounts for like heart,green tripe, smelt, and so on.

This pan set up lets me have EVERYTHING I need to add to meals within arms reach. My main prep area is directly next to the stove which is on my left, on the right side I keep my knife or knives, cutting board, scale, and paper plate for random things I need to set down that I don't want to set directly on the counter. To the right of my main prep area is the sink and to the right of the sink is another countertop surface where I keep my containers that will end up in the freezer. I also like to keep a box of gloves in an easily accessible place in case I need to take a pair of gloves off for just a minute to do something like answer a phone call or see what mischief the dogs are getting themselves into. I mean...my dogs behave perfectly...all the time...yeah let's go with that.

Simple, clean easy. I know where my bulk food is going, I know where my casily accessible prep food is going, I know where I'm working, and I know where my sink and containers are.

Easy peasy.

The last part of the system is what order do you do things in. What do you add to your dog's meals first, second, and so on. I'll go over my exact process later in this chapter.

Alright, let's move on to the next meal prepping section, "Prep for Prepping".

Prep For Prepping

In this section I want to cover how to prepare for your prepping. It may seem like a lot of steps right now but once you do it a few times everything just melds together and becomes seamless. You won't have to make plans because you already know what they are, you know how much of what you need, how to prepare things, and so on. So let's talk about prepping for prepping.

When I say "prep for prepping" or "prepping for prepping" I just mean getting everything together so that you can get started. Let's go over everything that you are going to need to do your meal preps.These are in no particular order of importance, this is just everything you'll need.

Food

You are obviously going to need food to prep or you won't have anything to prep.

Scheduled Prep Time

You are going to want to set aside a particular time that you prep. This might be a regular time every other week or so when you know you'll have time or it may need to be more sporadic. It all depends on your personal schedule.

Entertainment

I use meal prep as a time to turn my brain off, put on some bluetooth headphones, and just listen to a movie on Netflix while I do something great for my dogs.

Consider doing the same and meal prep may become one of your favorite events.

Containers

These are the containers you will actually put your dog's food in that will go in the freezer.
Some people simply use ziploc bags but I recommend getting some actually plastic containers from a company like ziploc which is what we use.
Ziploc bags are not only awful for the environment but you are spending more money because you are constantly buying more. Invest a few bucks (way less than $20) for some good plastic, reusable containers. Name brand if possible since they tend to be stronger.

Utensils

This covers everything from your knives, kitchen shears, or scoops and spatulas if you're working with ground meats.

Cutting board or boards.

Cutting boards are obviously good for preventing your counter from getting chopped up but they are also good for simply keeping juices and your meat off the counter.
I recommend getting a few different sizes but if you're only going to get one get a big one. They are extremely inexpensive.

Freezer

All this food needs to go somewhere right? Get yourself a good freezer, used if necessary. In the beginning you can start off with the freezer that's attached to your fridge but the sooner you can get a designated "dog food" freezer the better. They can be extremely cheap if you get them used and both stand up freezers and chest freezers work great.

I prefer upright freezers because they're easier on your back and their design makes it easier to see what's in them. For example, we got our full size upright freezer for $30 used off of a local yard sale group on Facebook and it's been running perfectly for years.

Gloves

Some would say this isn't a necessity and that you can just handle the meat. While they are right in the aspect that you CAN do that, I highly recommend and prefer using gloves.
It's more sanitary for obvious reasons, it's safer because if you get a good latex or latex alternative box of gloves they give you a better grip and wet knives,
and you leave less messes all over the place because if you need to do something like quickly grab your cell phone to answer a call you don't have to choose between missing the call or grabbing your cell phone with bloody hands. Just slip your gloves off and answer the call.

Food scale

A scale is necessary if you are going to do this whole thing accurately and they are VERY inexpensive. I have been using an $11 scale that measures oz, grams, and milliliters that I got off of Amazon for years.

Separation Containers

You'll need to have some pans, cookie sheets, or large dog bowls to put your food in next to your main prep area. This will allow you quick access to the food you need. You don't even need to buy new stuff for this, just use the kitchen items you already have around.

Sanitation Items

We'll go over sanitation in detail later in this chapter but you are going to need simple clean up items like paper towels, and disinfectant wipes or spray.

Reference Material

When you are just starting out it's a good idea to just have some sticky notes or information written down on a notepad close by. These sticky notes should have things on them like the bone content percentages of the meaty bones you'll be using that day, and total amounts you'll be prepping that day. Meaning X oz. of muscle meat, X oz. of bone, X oz. of liver, X oz. of non-liver organ. This way you don't have to memorize everything and you can simply refer to your lists if you have to.

The rest of your prepping prep is simply going to be putting everything in it's place so it's ready to go. Make sure your food is defrosted and ready to work with. Make sure all of your containers are out and ready for food. Make sure your utensils are good to go including making sure your knives are sharp. Make sure you have a box of gloves out and easily accessible. Set up your main prep area with your cutting board and scale and get those headphones on because it's time to get prepping!

In to the next meal prepping section we will actually go through the exact process I use when I'm meal prepping so you have something to model your meal prepping process from.

Meal Prepping Full Walk Through

In this section I want to cover the meat of this whole meal prepping topic…ok that was a lame joke. In this example I'll walk you through what I DO when preparing prey model style meals. These steps however can be EASILY modified to fit whatever raw feeding model you've chosen. But seriously, let's get right to it. I'm going to walk you through EVERYTHING I do for my meal preps. This is assuming that preps for preps have already been done. Everything is out and in it's proper place and ready to go.

I'm going to explain preparing a meal for my approximately 80 lb. German Shepherd Horus. Horus has always been a slim dog and does not require high feeding percentages to maintain his weight. This constantly changes as time goes on and he grows. "Observe and adjust." So he gets approximately 1.75% of his body weight. This amounts to 1.4 lbs or 22.5 oz. per day. Again, these numbers fluctuate from time to time depending on the time of year, his current weight, exercise, and so on. I'll say it again, "Observe and adjust."

Here is what that 22.5 oz a day looks like following the 80/10/5/5 equation. I'll need 17 oz of muscle meat or the 80%, 3 oz of bone (this is higher than the actual 10% because my dogs need a little bit more than 10%), and 1.25 oz of liver and non-liver organ or "the 5%" & "the other 5%".

In this meal we will be including ostrich liver, beef spleen, green tripe, turkey heart, turkey gizzards, and pork ribs for bone content.

Step #1 - Entertainment

Get those headphones on and put on your favorite show.

Step #2 - Gloves

Put on a pair of gloves, it's time to get started.

Step #3 - Organs / The 5% & Other 5%

Organs come first because they are something that is so much easier to cut when they are colder/partially frozen as opposed to getting closer to room temperature. A partially frozen organ is

1000x easier to cut up and handle. So at the "peak of coldness" I will cut them first.

For both the liver and non-liver organ I will need approx. 1.25 oz. Which one you do first doesn't really matter just complete one before moving on to the other. For example, if I can fit 10 containers on my counter (which I can) I will cut up 10 meals worth of the liver or non-liver organ and put those into the containers. Then I will repeat the process with the other organ.

To weigh the organ I will simply turn on my food scale, place a plate or container of some kind on top of the scale and weigh out the 1.25 oz. Make sure you zero out or "tare" your scale after you put the plate or container on the scale. All scales come with instructions on doing this.

Now all 10 meals have organ and I can move on.

Step #4 - Fill Prep Food Pans

Now I will fill up all of my pans that I am keeping next to my main prep area. This could involve cutting down racks of ribs into individual ribs, cutting meat down into the sizes my dogs need, breaking up a bag of tripe, cutting up bigger hearts like beef and pig hearts into smaller pieces, and so on.

Remember that you should have 4 fairly large pans or containers for this food. One for organs that you already used, one for your bone content like ribs, one for your main 80% meats like gizzards or pork chunks, and one for 80% category foods that you'll use less of like green tripe and hearts.

Now you may be asking why I don't do this process back in Step #3 but again, that's because I want to cut the organs while they are still as cold as possible to make my job easier. You may choose to make Step #4 part of YOUR Step #3 and that's completely fine. I'm explaining it this way because I told you I was going to explain exactly how I do things during meal prep.

Step #5 - Bone Content / The 10%

Now that I have everything I need to finish the meals put into those pans I can continue putting the meal together and the next item on our list is bone.

Remembering that I need 3 oz of bone I will weigh the pork rib. Again I'll do this by placing the rib on the plate I used to weigh the organs that is on the scale.

To easily explain this process let's say that the pork rib weighs just over 9 oz.

Because I know that pork ribs are approx. ⅓ or 33% bone, I know that this single rib takes care of my bone needs and also provides me with 6 oz of muscle meat so I'll put that into a container and repeat the process for each container. Just like the organs, do all the bone for all the containers on the counter at once.

Don't over stress being exact here.

Most of the foods you will use for bone like ribs, necks, turkey wings, etc...will be generally the same size and weight but if you come across a 10 oz rib then don't worry about it and just move on keeping the rest of your measurements the same. A small difference like that isn't going to do any harm. Again, don't stress being exact.

Let's review really quick to make sure you are following along on the math because a lot of people struggle with it.

I started off needing 22.5 oz total of food per meal. Then I added 2.5 oz of organ between the ostrich liver and beef spleen to the containers (1.25 oz. each) leaving me with 20 oz of food still needing to be added.

Then I added a 9 oz rib which was approx 3 oz. of bone and 6 oz of meat leaving me with 11 oz of food still needing to be added.

Because I know I need 17 oz total of meat and 6 of it has already been taken care of by the rib, I know that the rest of the meal will be meat. "The 80%".

Step #6 - Meat Content / The 80%

Now comes the last addition to the meal which is going to be meat or the 80% which again we now need 11 oz of.

At this point with the food I am using for this particular example I will add a small handful of green tripe that is typically 1 - 2 oz, a piece of heart that is also around 1 oz, and then finish up with my main meat source which in this example is turkey gizzards.

There is no need to stress the exact amounts. For example, if you need 8 oz of turkey gizzards and the scale says 9 oz don't try and cut 1 oz of turkey gizzard away from one of the gizzards. Now if the smallest amount of gizzards you have available makes the scale say 16 oz then yes, use your knife and cutting board to get as close to 8 oz as possible.

The whole point here is to get as close as you can to the needed amount but don't give yourself a headache trying to cut away minute amounts of food that aren't going to have any impact on your dog.

I'll repeat this process for the remaining 9 containers. Now, as far as adding food to my 10 original containers goes I'm completely done!

Step #7 - Containers in the freezer

Now that the containers are full, take your disposable gloves off, chuck em, put lids on your containers, take a picture of them and tag @dogdadofficial and @rawfeeding101 on Instagram of course, and then stack them in the freezer.

Step #8 - Repeat steps 2 -7

Repeat these steps until you run out of food, space in your freezer, or containers. If you had multiple sources for things like meat, bone, and organs, consider doing one full set of meals, in this case 10, with one group of foods and then one full set of meals with a different group of foods. If you do happen to have multiple sources and can make different meals consider stacking each group together in the freezer.

One of the meals on the right or on one shelf, and the other meal on the left or a separate shelf.
This way as you are going through the meals you've created throughout the week you can pull from one shelf or stack one day and the other the next day. This allows you to maintain variety not only as far as what foods you are feeding is concerned, but also on a day by day basis.

Sometimes dogs will get picky and start refusing food if they have the same meal over and over again which can happen if you prepped a month's worth of food.

Step #9 - Put excess food away

This will be necessary if you happen to run out of freezer space, containers, or run out of a food group that you need like liver or bone content but still have plenty of meat available.

Step #10 - CleanUp

The next and final meal prepping section will cover step #10, the cleanup process.

Congratulations!

Once you get through these steps you have successfully completed your meal prepping. Now all you have to do to feed your dogs a balanced diet on a daily basis is pull it out of the freezer to defrost, add any supplements you are feeding, if any at meal time, and feed away.

Most people prefer to pull it out the night before and put it in the fridge to defrost so it's ready the next day. If you're going to feed like me and feed once a day in the evening, you can just pull it out in the morning, set it on the counter somewhere, and feed it before it reaches room temperature.

P.S. Once a day feedings are only acceptable for adults, never feed a puppy under 12 months old only once a day. Alright on to the last meal prepping section, cleanup and sanitation.

Cleanup & Sanitation

One of the biggest concerns anti-raw people harp on and that prospective raw feeders worry about is one of the human family members getting sick.
Without proper cleanup and sanitation this CAN be a concern but with some simple, easy to follow clean up steps we can avoid with near certainty.
Like my good friend and operator of keepthetailwagging.com Kimberly Morris Gauthier says, "If you can prepare and feed a turkey dinner, you can feed raw."

Cleanup and sanitation really is super simple and doesn't require a whole lot of effort but is super effective. Here's what I do and what I recommend you do.

Step #1
Discard any remaining containers that your food came in like plastic bags and so on. Essentially, throw away the trash.

Step #2

Place all your pans, bowls, utensils, cutting boards, etc.... in the sink to be washed. Ideally wash them right there and then. If that's not possible, do it as soon as possible. If you are lucky enough to have a dishwasher, rinse them and place them in the dishwasher.

Step #3

Dry off all of the surfaces that you and/or the raw food interacted with paper towels. This includes tables, counters, the stove, food scale, EVERYTHING. You need to get all the juices, blood, and so on off the surfaces before you can sanitize them.

Step #4

Sanitize EVERYTHING that you dried off that you and/or the raw food interacted with.
Again, this includes EVERYTHING. Your food scale, tables, counters, stove, sink, faucets, everything. You can either use a spray cleaner of some kind and paper towels or disinfectant wipes. Name brand doesn't matter in this case, they all work just as well in my experience. Regardless of whether you choose to get spray or wipes make sure that you are using one that claims it "kills 99.9% of germs and bacteria".

If you are uncomfortable with chemical cleaners like that explore other options like seventh generation brand cleaners. I've used them from time to time and never seen any negative effects or rather I should say LACK of effectiveness but do your own research to see if these natural alternatives will be effective enough to make you comfortable.

Step #5

Throw away all of the paper towels or sanitary wipes, then wash your hands and take out the trash so you aren't spreading the germs to your door knobs, etc…

Step #6

Put a brand new bag in your trash can and yet again, **WASH YOUR HANDS**.

WASH YOUR HANDS

WASH YOUR HANDS

WASH YOUR HANDS

Chapter 6

Common Issues & What You Can Do About Them

Your Dog Refuses Their Raw Food

The first common problem I want to talk about is when dog's refuse to eat their raw food during the transition. It's a lot more common than you'd think so let's dive in.

As human beings we often think that if a dog is offered a plate of raw, meaty goodness they would dive right in and there's little chance we'd be able to stop them even if we wanted to.
Now for a lot of new raw feeders that is absolutely true. My german shepherds never had any problems with this.

Horus had already had tastes of raw by the time we got him from the breeder at 9 weeks old so he was easy peasy. Wolken on the other hand was 10 months old when we adopted him and had been on kibble his whole life. The first thing we fed him was a skinless, bone in chicken breast and he dove right in like a natural...which he of course is.

These success stories are unfortunately not what every new raw feeder experiences. Some dogs have been on kibble for so long that they are quite literally addicted to it. On the other hand, some dogs are just set in their ways and refuse to see anything other than their precious pellets as food.

So what can people that experience these kinds of problems do to get their dog to finally accept the idea of raw. In my opinion there are two main options that can be effective and safe.

Option 1. A 24 Hour Fast

In the transition portion of the book you will see that I recommend a 24 hour fast between the last kibble meal and the first raw meal. There are several reasons for that but we'll discuss it then.

In this circumstance the 24 hour fast serves as an incentive to eat the raw food because the dog is hungry. This means that the kibble addicts and picky, "stuck in their ways" dogs are more likely to give the raw food a try and hopefully enjoy it.

Now I know you may be thinking, "Oh I could never not feed my dog for a full 24 hours, I just couldn't do it." and I totally understand.

You don't want your dog going hungry which is completely understandable but I want you to consider something. When a dog has diarrhea or vomiting one of the most commonly vet recommended and effective solutions is a 24 hour fast from food. NOT WATER...that's important. Never deny a dog water.

With this in mind, you can take comfort in knowing that it's not going to be harmful in any way to your dog and you are going to have a harder time with it than your dog is. There are of course exceptions to this if your dog has a medical condition that can be negatively impacted by fasting. Please speak with your vet if that is the case for you.

So if the dog refuses the raw food, fast them for 24 hours and give it another try. If they still refuse then give them their kibble and try again with raw the next day.

Option 2. Mixing & Slowly Increasing

If your dog refuses the raw food and you've tried the 24 hour fast method without success, try option 2 which is essentially just adding raw food to the kibble. Start by slowly increasing the amount of raw and decreasing the kibble until you reach full raw with kibble sprinkled on top and eventually full raw.

It is very important that you do not feed bones while you are going through this mixing phase.
Kibble impacts the PH of a dog's stomach acid in a way that may leave it less capable of properly preparing bone for digestion in the small intestine.

So if you are forced to resort to this method of transitioning, start "Week 1" of the transition AFTER you have successfully made it through the mixing phase.

So there you have it. A couple of easy and simple solutions to help convince that kibble addicted or picky dog transition to a raw diet.

Poop Problems

In this section I want to cover another common problem that a lot of new raw feeders experience and that's "weird poops".

Let's get right to it.

The perfect poop that we are looking for as raw feeders is the solid, easy to pick up, chocolate to dark chocolate colored poops. Often times though even with fully transitioned dogs, poops that don't match that description can occur.
Here's some of those "weird poops" and what you can do about them.

Diarrhea

Diarrhea can be caused by a plethora of things. Adjusting to new foods, stress, genuine illness from an infection of some kind, or an everyday upset stomach. Over the years I have spoken with several vet techs who have told me that the most common and effective treatment for a one time bout of diarrhea is a 24 hour fast. It gives the body a chance to eliminate whatever is causing the issue in their system by devoting the vast majority of it's energy towards that purpose instead of spending energy on digesting more food that could make the situation worse.

It's not unlike human beings being sick and not having much of an appetite if they have one at all. The body doesn't have an appetite because it's trying to devote it's energy to the problem.

Dehydration can cause a lot of damage and it can happen in an extremely short amount of time. With that in mind, seriously consider a vet visit if your dog has continued diarrhea for more than 24 hours especially if it's accompanied by vomiting, your dog stops drinking water, bloating occurs which will often be accompanied by major gas, or your dog exhibits unusual behavior like being lethargic or just not acting like themselves.

Again, dehydration causes lots of problems and it causes them fast. If your dog exhibits the behaviors or symptoms I just listed I urge you to consider a visit with your veterinarian as soon as possible.

Mucus Poops

Mucus is exactly what it sounds like, a "mucusy" type substance that can either cover an entire piece of poop or smaller sections of the poop.

A lot of raw feeders experience this in the first few days to weeks of raw feeding and then it goes away on it's own as the dog's body adjusts. Most often though mucus is simply caused by an upset stomach so if you have a dog that is experiencing mucus covered poops and is already transitioned to a raw diet try, again, a 24 hour fast. This again give the body an opportunity to put all of it's energy towards fixing the problem.

If the problem still continues consider a vet visit to make sure your dog hasn't contracted a bacterial infection from something like dirty water or another dog they met or encountered during that walk the other day or parasites from similar sources.

Black Poops

Black poops are are typically softer and can be accompanied by a bit of runniness. Black poops can easily be caused by too much organ in the diet but can also be caused by bleeding farther back in the digestive system which is a real issue.

If you have a dog with black poops consider going a day without organs and seeing if the black poops continue. If they don't, great. Just reduce your organ amounts slightly. If they do continue, highly consider a vet visit.

Bloody Poops

Bloody poop is never a good thing. At the very least your dog cut a minor cut or abrasion of some kind somewhere in or near their rectum, or anus which is obviously not fun for them.
On the more serious end of the spectrum something very serious is happening and your dog is passing blood.

If you see blood in your dog's stool it's most certainly time for a vet visit as soon as possible, possibly even an emergency visit depending on the amount of blood.

Constipation

As raw feeders we most typically see constipation after a dog has had too much bone. It can also be caused by a lack or excess of fiber in the diet.

If your dog is having a hard time pooping make sure they are getting plenty of water and get them moving. Exercise helps "Get things moving", literally.

Whatever you do, do not give your dog laxatives that were meant for human beings without working with your vet, preferably a holistic one.

If you have a dog that has not had a movement for several days it's time to go to a veterinarian, period.

I hope that this list of common poop issues that raw feeders face has been helpful. Like everything else, be observant, apply at home remedies when it's appropriate, and if necessary don't hesitate on a vet visit. Better safe than sorry...truly.

Vomiting Issues

In this section I want to cover vomiting. Vomiting is something that a lot of dogs do randomly from time to time and does not necessarily indicate a problem that you should be concerned about.
Let's talk about a few different kinds of vomiting. Hunger pukes, regurgitation, grassy pukes, and vomiting that should concern you.

Hunger Pukes

Hunger pukes are caused when a dog anticipates food but does not get it. The basic science of this is as follows.

When a dog anticipates food whether that's a treat or a meal the dog starts to produce saliva and starts to secrete gastric acid, more commonly known as stomach acid in their stomach.
This stomach acid is very strong. If the dog does not use that secreted acid by consuming food it can cause the dog to throw up.

Typically when a dog hunger pukes it appears as light to dark yellow foamy liquid. To avoid hunger pukes maintain a regular feeding schedule. Everything from when you pull your food out of the fridge or freezer to what time of day you feed meals.

If you have a dog that seems to be constantly having hunger pukes consider increasing the amount of times you are feeding per day.

Regurgitation

Regurgitation can happen for a few different reasons. It could be that the dog ate too fast and the body is essentially saying, "Whoa, too much too fast. Give it another try." It could also be that the dog didn't chew well and the body is again saying, "Give it another try."

If you have a dog that is eating too fast you can try special bowls that can be found all over the internet designed for fast eaters to help them slow down.

If you have a dog that is not chewing very well you can try feeding larger pieces of food that are partially frozen or you can hold food like chicken drumsticks, etc…which forces them to chew on it. This is obviously not recommended for dogs with food aggression but you should consult a professional about those problems.

If your dog DOES regurgitate their food you can either clean it up or let them eat it again.

As gross as it sounds, I recommend the latter.

Your dog's mouth already has vomit in it from throwing the food up so all you will be doing by cleaning it up without giving them the opportunity to eat it is wasting the food. If your dog regurgitates on the carpet that may be a different story and you may want to at least transfer the big pieces to a hard surface and then clean the rest up immediately.

Grassy Pukes

Some dogs that eat grass will throw up afterwards but not all dogs will. Not even dogs with a history of doing this will always vomit after eating grass.

Unless your dog eats grass and vomits over and over again and can not keep water down then you should be fine. If however they ARE doing all of that, then it's time for a vet visit. This is because of what I've talked about before, the dangers of dehydration.

When Vomiting Should Concern You

There are some overall signs that can indicate a real problem when it comes to vomiting. If you notice any of these symptoms they may be cause for concern and you should highly consider a vet visit.

When I say "Highly recommend" I mean I'm not going to tell you when to go to the vet but if my dogs were showing these symptoms I'd absolutely be going to the vet.

These signs or symptoms are:
- Vomiting that happens over and over which is preventing the dog from keeping down water, especially if this is accompanied by diarrhea
- Blood is in the dog's vomit
- Vomiting that occurs after a large amount of what looks like hiccups accompanied by licking of the lips & Vomit that is accompanied or followed by a bloated/distended stomach.
- The mother of all emergencies.

This last one, vomiting and a visually bloated stomach has been called "the mother of all emergencies" and can kill within hours. This last symptom can be the sign that the bloated stomach has rotated trapping gas and food and has also been cut off from it's blood supply.

As you can see, vomit can commonly be caused by a large variety of things. Some harmless to nearly harmless, some so life threatening that it can kill in hours. The best advice I can give you is to be aware of the difference between the two and if you ever think your dog is experiencing a serious problem, get them to the vet.

You'll either be told everything is fine and you overreacted, or you'll have potentially saved your dog's life.

Both sound like a win to me.

Chapter 7

The Transition

BEFORE YOU GET STARTED...

Before getting started with the transition phase please make sure that you have read chapters 1 through 6. It's critical that you educate yourself before starting so **PLEASE** read all of those chapters before you get started.

I DO NOT recommend you just skip to the transition steps.

You WILL Be Nervous

When it comes to the transition you WILL be nervous so let's talk about that for a minute.

Sorry, but it's the truth. You ARE going to be nervous. Just breathe. Remember what we talked about earlier in this book. You've been programmed over the years to believe that commercial food is the only safe way to feed your dog. You've probably even seen some companies vilify raw feeding to protect their own profit margins. More importantly, remember the powerful, efficient, and instinctual carnivore that your dog is. With zero to little effort and patience on your part they will remember what it is to eat meat and will dive right in.

Know you are doing the right thing, remember that THOUSANDS and THOUSANDS and THOUSANDS of other dog owners have already made the switch with their dogs and those dogs and are living happier, healthier, hopefully longer lives.

You've done the responsible thing by educating yourself BEFORE starting on a raw diet. I've shared with you some of the common issues you may see and what you can do about them. I've told you how you can prepare meals ahead of time to make your life easier. I've taught you some basics about overcoming mental barriers and dealing with difficult situations.

You can do this...

Don't second guess yourself and just do it and again, remember that you aren't alone. You can always join me and my community in the Raw Feeding 101 - Learn To Feed Raw" Facebook group for support.

It's time to get your dog started on a raw diet.

How This Transition Is Set Up

In this section I want to tell you how the transition phase of the book is set up and how you should use it. First let's talk about how the transition is set up.

The transition you will be going through using this book is going to utilize the slow transition method as opposed to the balanced from the start method. They are two very different transition methods. Both with their pros and cons. Some people prefer a balanced from the start approach.

Balanced From The Start

A balanced from the start approach is exactly what it sounds like. You are balancing the diet from the very first meal/ There is no introduction period it's everything all at once. Meat, bones, liver, other organs, everything. The only benefit in my personal opinion with this method is that everything the dog needs comes all at once so there is no period where the dog is missing out on anything. Which if I'm honest is a pretty big benefit…

The con of this transition method is that it simply doesn't go well far too often. I can't tell you how many times I have seen someone go from kibble to a balanced from the start and have a terrible experience.

Now I'm not saying it can't work but more often than not in my experience it's simply too much for the dog's system to handle. Too many new things all at the same time and the body doesn't know what to do with it. It'd be like if you went from eating McDonald's and processed food everyday to a high fiber, all organic etc...diet. Even though the food is better for you, you'd end up sitting on the toilet for a long time because your body just didn't know what to do with all of it.

Now let's talk about the slow transition approach.

Slow Transitions

The slow transition approach is again what you will be learning in this book. The slow transition approach introduces one thing at a time and allows the dog's body to adjust to that new food item before moving on to the next food item.
In this chapter I've broken down the transition period into 4 weeks or steps. As each week or step passes you will be adding another piece of puzzle or in this case a new food item to your dog's diet.

At the end of the 4th step you will be feeding some form of the 80/10/5/5 formula! With this slow approach you get the major pro of giving your dog the best possible chance of acclimating to a raw diet without any type of digestive upset like diarrhea or vomiting.

The con of this approach is that there is a 3-4 week period where your dog's diet is not balanced with the 80/10/5/5 formula.

Now let's talk about how to use this transition properly

How To Use This Transition

       I said before that this transition is broken into 4 weeks or steps, that being said, you should only move on to the next week or step if your dog is handling the current week or step well. To clarify a little bit here, I say week OR step because sometimes some dogs need longer to adjust to a particular set so sometimes the time you spend on a step may not be exactly a week.

When your dog is ready to move to the next step will mostly be determined by your dog's poop. If your dog's poop is not mostly solid and mostly chocolate colored you should continue with the current week or step for another few days to a full week.

For example, if week 1 goes well but in week 2 you are having trouble getting solid poops, don't just go to week 3 just because you hit the next week on the calendar. The whole idea is to give your dog's body time to adjust to the new food coming in. If you add in more new things before it's handling the current new foods well then you could just be making things worse. Listen to your dog's body, it will tell you when it's ready if you listen.

Let's also touch on how much to feed during the transition while you are not feeding all portions of the 80/10/5/5 formula. In the original version of my online course I did not clarify this very well so I want to make sure I am very specific here.

During the transition only feed the amount of the items you have added to the diet at whatever point you are at. I know that's confusing so let me lay it out.

For example, during the first 2 weeks you will only be feeding the 80% muscle meat, and 10% bone portion of the formula.

So if the calculator included with the purchase of this book tells you to feed 17 oz of muscle meat, 2.25 oz. off bone, 1.25 oz of liver and 1.25 oz of other organ, only feed the 17 oz. Of muscle meat and the 2.25 oz of bone during the first 2 weeks/steps.

Meaning the total amount of food you will be feeding during the first 2 steps would be 19.25 oz.

When you hit week or step 3 and start adding liver, you'll be feeding the 17 oz of meat, 2.25 oz. of bone, and 1.25 oz of liver.

Meaning the total amount of food would then be 20.5 oz.

When you add in your non-liver organ at the beginning of week or step 4 you'll be feeding the 17 oz of meat, 2.25 oz. of bone, 1.25 oz of liver, and the 1.25 oz of non-liver organ which is the full 80/10/5/5 formula or in this example 21.75 oz.

The whole idea is that you are only using the parts of the formula that you are currently feeding based on where you are in the transition.

In summary, the transition method used in this book will be a slow transition method that allows the body to adjust to new things, one thing at a time and you shouldn't be moving onto the next week/step until things are going well.

Figuring Out How Much To Feed

SO, how much should you feeding? Now that is a good question isn't it? How much DO you feed? Maybe you have a 12 lb pomeranian, maybe you have a 83 lb GSD like me. There is obviously going to be a massive difference in how much to feed to a 12 lb pom vs an 83 lb GSD.

So how do you figure it out?

Well it's actually extremely simple. I have a calculator spreadsheet for you which is included with this book. You'll have to download it because it is a digital calculator but you can find details on how to do that in the "Online & Downloadable Resources" section at the end of this book.

That calculator will allow you to enter your dog's weight and it will automatically tell you how much meat, bone, liver and other organs to feed on a daily basis. It even has multiple tabs so you can get daily amounts with multiple dogs all at the same time.

It's essentially going to spit out the "Secret Formula" numbers that we talked about earlier in the book. The 80/10/5/5.

Also, to make sure I am taking care of my readers in and out of the U.S. there are 2 different versions available. One version that works with pounds and ounces and one version that works with grams and kilograms.

Pretty simple right? Well it is! It's important to remember though that these are starting or base guidelines. You may need to adjust these numbers for your dog WITHIN REASON.

Remember my statement earlier? "Observe and Adjust"

Your dog might require as an example, a slightly higher amount of bone than the average dog. Maybe they'll need a little bit less. I mentioned this earlier in the meal prepping section of the book but here is a personal example. I should be feeding 2.25 oz of bone daily but I have to feed 3 oz+ to ensure I get solid poops for both of my GSDs.

The point is that while these numbers (80/10/5/5) are an AMAZING starting point, they aren't the etched in stone law that you should stay on permanently.

"Observe and Adjust"

Another flashback to earlier in the book, a student of the original version of my online course worked with a holistic vet and had to take their bone % up to 24% before the dog would balance out. This isn't typical and the percentage was reduced after that but the point is that no two dogs are the same and you should adjust when you see the need to.

If you are going to be feeding premade or complete grinds you are obviously not going to have total control over these numbers and will have follow the steps I described in the "Feeding Grinds & Premades & What You Need To Know" section of this book.

If you are going to be feeding BARF or including fruits and vegetables into your dog's diet, I personally recommend starting off with this prey model approach, (or the "Secret Formula" as I've called it throughout the book) and then do further research into how you would like to incorporate fruits and vegetables.

I talked a lot about fruits and veggies being added to the diet earlier in the book so refer back to that section and again do more research as the amount of fruits and veggies that some people add varies greatly by as much as 20%.

Also, for those that are concerned about getting bone % right, there is an additional bone calculator included with the book that I will describe in more detail in another section.

Another important aspect of how much to feed is whether you are going to balance the diet on a daily basis or if you are going to balance over time. While balancing over time works out great for others I highly suggest you balance on a daily basis until you get a hold of things. It's just one less thing you have to remember and worry about. Less stress for you means less stress for your dog. It also makes things like meal prepping SIGNIFICANTLY easier like we already discussed earlier in the book.

I have to mention one last thing that trips up a lot of beginners and that is the "How many times a day do I feed?" question.

How Often To Feed

How many times a day you feed a day is completely up to you unless you have a puppy, they should be fed no less than 3 times a day. I'll talk about puppies later in this chapter. For the adult dogs, feeding 1 meal a day, 2 meals a day, it doesn't really matter.

Just divide the daily amount of food you should be feeding into however many meals you choose. The meals themselves don't have to be balanced individually. So if you choose to feed twice a day feel free to give your bone content in one meal and everything else in a second meal, and so on.

So the bottomline is figure out how much your dog weighs, use the daily amount calculator that has been provided to you, divide your total amount of food by how many meals a day you are feeding, and adjust where necessary as you observe your dog overtime.

Getting The Right Amount Of Bone

In this section I am going to tell you how to use the Raw Feeding 101 - Bone Content Calculator spreadsheet. This way you'll be able to figure out how much bone and meat is in what bone content foods you are feeding so that you can provide the correct amount of bone in your dog's diet.

Step 1. Weigh the food item that you are working with.

This could be a turkey wing, duck neck, or in this example we'll be using a pork rib.
Enter the total weight of that pork rib in either ounces or grams depending on what you are most comfortable with in the "Enter food weight:" section of the bone content calculator.

This section is marked "Step 1"

In this example we are going to say that this pork rib weighs 9 ounces so I would type "9" in the "Enter food weight" section of the calculator.

Step 2. Find the approximate percentage of bone for the food you are working with.

You can do this by looking at great sources online like Perfectly Rawsome. I use the bone content guide at the following address on a regular basis: perfectlyrawsome.com/bone. In this example again we are going to use pork ribs that are approximately 33% bone. Enter that number into the "Enter average bone%" section of the bone content calculator that is marked as "Step 2".

You don't need to enter the actual % sign, just the number. In other words you would enter "33" not "33%". So in this example I would type 33 and then click anywhere else on the bone content calculator to activate the automatic calculation.

Step 3. Observe your results.

In this example after clicking outside of the "Step 2" section your rounded results will populate in the "Bone Weight" and "Meat Weight" sections of the bone content calculator. With the example of a pork rib that weighs 9 oz at approximately 33% bone, our rounded amounts are 3 oz of bone and 6 ounces of content.

Step 4. Get Creative.

At this point you can use the calculator to do a lot of different things.

For example, if you find that the pork ribs you get weigh anywhere from 9 - 11 ounces you can do the calculations for all of those different weights and write them down for reference later. This way you'll have accurate bone content amounts and you won't have to use the calculator for every piece of bone content you feed.

Consider keeping a small notebook or spreadsheet on your computer with different results for the most common bone content sources you feed.

Changes In Water Consumption

This section is going to be very short because it's only about one main idea that tends to concern a lot of few raw feeders and that is a change in how much water your dog drinks after the transition vs pre-transition.

In most cases when dogs are switched over to raw they almost immediately start drinking less water. Understandably, this immediately concerns pet parents because they know their dog needs water and they are used to them drinking so much more.

Water, moisture, etc... is key in every aspect of your dog's body, function, digestion and so on.
The starches and dry nature of kibble soaks up and uses a lot of the water in the body to aid in the digestion of the kibble which causes the dogs to drink a lot more water. With a raw diet this "soaking up" of water from the body to aid in digestion and more is much less severe because the food itself is packed full of moisture. The muscle meat, bones, liver, organs, and even fruits and veggies all contain high levels of moisture.

Because the dog is no longer having to make up for all the water the kibble is soaking up, the dog starts drinking a lot less water because they simply don't need to.

Now please, don't ever deny your dog water just because you made the switch, always provide a ton of fresh water for when your dog needs it.

The purpose of this section was to tell you to expect a decline in water consumption after the switch so that you do not worry and think something is wrong.

Alright, on to the next part of the transition section of the book.

Your dog's first...raw...meal.

(Queue the "I'm so excited!" song.)

Your Dog's First Raw Meal & Week 1/ Step 1

In this section I want to talk about what you need to do before your first meal, feeding your first meal, and the rest of the first week.

LET'S DO THIS THING!

Let me first start by clarifying that this transition method will be specifically for adult dogs. I will address transitioning puppies in another section. There are important differences.

Bone In - White Meat Protein

The first thing you need to do is to obtain a bone in, white meat source. In this slow approach transition method you will be starting with a bone in, white meat protein. You need to keep things bland and simple at first.

Chicken is ideal and is the easiest to get your hands on but turkey or rabbit will work also if you happen to raise them or it's readily available in your area. If your dog already has a known allergy to chicken, start with the next cheapest white meat source you have available to you and try chicken again after your dog is transitioned.

Side Note

Sometimes dogs that have allergies to chicken based kibbles can handle raw chicken just fine. If chicken is your only option you can still try it and see what happens. If at all possible, I recommend starting with turkey or rabbit if you have a dog that may have a chicken allergy or intolerance and THEN try giving them raw chicken after the transition. This way you won't have to wonder if the issues you potentially see are from the transition or the chicken, you'll know it was the chicken.

Red meat is simply too rich for a lot of dogs to start with so don't roll that dice because you might lose. Start with bone in, white meat.

Remember to only feed the amount of food of what you are feeding at the moment. Again. that means that during the first week, use the daily amount calculator provided with the book and only feed the muscle meat and bone weight/amount. Don't feed additional meat or bones to make up for the liver and other organ, just leave them out of the total weight/amount of the meal for now like we talked about earlier.

Next You'll need to Decide Where You Will Feed

Wherever it is that you decide to feed keep a few things in mind. The area you choose should be easily cleaned and sanitized, and it should be consistent. Don't feed in the kitchen one day, the back room with hardwood floors another day, etc... It's perfectly fine to feed outside sometimes and inside others BUT, make sure you have consistency.

In other words, pick ONE spot that you feed in the house and ONE spot that you feed outside to the best of your abilities. Dogs like predictability as much as anyone else.

I would also recommend putting your dog's leash around a stationary object and putting them on leash when feeding outside if you do not have a fenced yard.

Next, The 24 Hour Fast

Some say this isn't necessary, some say it is. I will tell you this though. Every dog that I have owned myself and every dog's owner I have personally coached into feeding a raw diet has put their dog through a 24 hour fast between the dog's last kibble or canned food meal and the dog's first raw meal. To this day, it has served me, the dogs, and their owners VERY well.

I truly believe this is because the digestive system is cleared and ready to accept new food. Now, I know a lot of people that never put their dog through a 24 hour fast and things went well for them during the transition. I can only tell you about my personal experiences and the experiences of those I've worked with.

Another, more scientifically backed up reason to do a 24 hour fast is PH in the dog's stomach.
Commercial food like kibble interferes with the dog's stomach acid's natural ph levels. The stomach acid breaks down calcium in bones and prepares the bones for digestion in the small intestine.

The 24 hour fast gives the body a chance to make some changes to that ph level. It's not perfect but again, all I can do is provide information on what my students and I have experienced.

I HIGHLY HIGHLY HIGHLY recommend you do a 24 hour fast before the first meal. Keep in mind though, this section is for adult dogs and not puppies.

A Day When You Are Home

I have found that it can be EXTREMELY helpful for you to have the day of your first meal off from work with no other plans. This allows you to feed the first meal, preferably in the morning, and then spend the day monitoring your dog. You'll be less stressed, worry less, and in turn enjoy the experience a lot more.

First Meal

Yes! It is finally time to feed your first meal! SOO exciting!

It is TIME to dive in. You just need to do it.

I know you may be nervous, heck maybe you're so stoked you can hardly wait. Either way, it's time. I'm not going to make this part particularly long because it's extremely simple. You know what you need to know, you're in a good mindset, it's time to begin.

Feed...your...dog's...first...raw...meal. Do it. Go on I'll wait.

If you're reading all the transition sections before starting then come back to this section if you get nervous about your first meal.

So what do you do for the rest of week 1? Like I said before, you need to start bland to allow your dog time to adjust. Until your dog is having firm, chocolate colored poops feed only white meat and the bone of that white meat protein source. I recommend doing this for a full week even if you never see loose poops.

If at the end of the first week your dog is still experiencing some slightly loose poops increase the bone content a little bit until you get firm, chocolate colored poops.

When this happens, move on to the next step.

However, remember what I talked about in the "How the transition is set up" section, don't move on from any particular week or step until you have firm, chocolate colored poops.

Some dogs just take longer to adjust, it's as simple as that. If you need some reassurance feel free to join my FB Group "Raw Feeding 101 - Learn To Feed Raw".

Week 2/ Step 2

In this section I want to address the 2nd week or 2nd step of your raw feeding journey. Whether it's the 2nd week or 2nd step is of course going to be determined by how well your dog adjusted to the 1st week or first step.

It's week or step 2, what now?

Once your dog has been on white meat and bone only for a week or more it's time to spice things up. It's time to introduce another protein source. A red meat protein source to be specific. Don't bother trying to find a bone in red meat source yet, keep using your bone in white protein source for your bone content.

Beef, pork, or even lamb will fit the bill for a red meat protein. Avoid elk, venison, antelope, and other large red meat animals that are typically hunted and not bought at the grocery store as these meats tend to upset the stomachs of dogs that are new to a raw diet. They tend to be EXTREMELY rich and can cause loose poops even for transitioned dogs having it for the first time.

Add a small amount of your chosen red meat protein and lead up to a 50% white meat, 50% red meat split in your dog's meals. This will introduce the new source in a gradual manner and give your dog time to accept it and adjust.

If your dog does well right off the bat you should be able to get to the 50/50 split by the end of a 7-day period. If it takes longer and you need to go into another week to do this then that is fine. Once you get firm, chocolate colored poops your dog has adjusted to the new red meat protein source.

If your dog adjusted by the end of week 2 or step 2, then move on to week or step 3. If your dog is taking a little bit longer to adjust that's completely fine and you should continue to feed this way until the end of the next week or until they adjust. At that point you can start "week 3" or step 3.

Week 3/ Step 3

In this section I want to talk about week or step 3. This tends to be the most difficult part of the transition for some dogs. Some dogs get through step 3 with no issues but if your dog is going to have issues it's probably going to be here.

So let's get to it.

Step 3 is potentially the most difficult step like I just mentioned. This step is a little bit difficult for the dog to adjust to. In step 3 you are going to be introducing liver.

Liver and organs in general are notorious for giving dogs loose stools in the beginning. That being said though, there are dogs with iron stomachs out there and things go off without a hitch. It's also helpful to start with the liver from a protein source you are already feeding. If you're feeding chicken and pork as an example, feed chicken or pork liver. Feeding turkey and beef? Try turkey or beef liver. You get the idea.

By doing this you aren't taking the additional risk of trying the liver from a new protein source that your dog could potentially have an intolerance or allergy for.

Like a lot of other things I've talked about in this book, you are going to want to start slow to give your dog the best chance of no loose stools. Start by adding 25% of the amount that the daily amount calculator you were provided says to feed.

For example, if it says to feed 1 oz. of liver feed then feed ¼ oz. or 0.25 oz if you're using a digital food scale which I highly recommend you do. When you see firm poops increase this amount to 50% of the calculated daily amount, then 75% and so on until you reach the full, calculated amount.

Keep in mind that this is most likely going to be the most difficult portion of the transition for you. Go as slow as you need to.

Only after you're feeding the full amount of liver recommended by the daily amount calculator should you move on to week/step 4.

Week 4/ Step 4

In this section we are going to talk about the final step, step 4 in the transition process.

Let's get started.

Your dog is eating meat, bone, and liver, now what?

Now that your dog is successfully eating it's full amount of liver without issues and you are seeing "holy grail" type poops which again are firm, brown, and easy to pick up, it's now time to add in non-liver organ.

Just like liver, start slow.

Because your dog is now eating one type of organ via the liver, this transition step should be easy but you are still introducing more new organ content. This increased organ content also comes with the potential risk of loose stools.

To avoid this, you want to start slowly just like you did with the liver. Also, just like the liver start by feeding 25% of the recommended amount that the daily amount calculator provided you and gradually work your way up to the full 100%

Again, go slow, go at your dog's body's pace and if loose stools occur more than once then reduce the amount just a little bit until poops firm up and then start increasing your feeding amount again.

That's it!!

That's the last step of the transition!

But...what to do now? You can't stop there...

Alright, on to the "Beyond week 4 section."

Beyond Week 4

CONGRATULATIONS!

You've completed the final steps of the initial transition. I am SO excited for you! Let's talk about what you should be doing as soon as you are done with the initial transition.

Now that you are done with the initial transition I want you to do one basic thing.

STEP UP YOUR GAME!

That's right step up your game and get better and better. Sure, you can get better equipment, buy a grinder and so on but I have two main things in mind when I say you should step up your game.

1. Start increasing your variety.

Now that you've made the transition with your white meat bone in protein, a red meat source, and your organs it's time to broaden your horizons. Start slowly introducing new proteins, new bone sources, new liver sources, and new non-liver organ sources.

Variety, variety, variety.

Variety is key. Use the "Introducing new proteins" section to do this and as always, start new things slowly.

But how are you going to provide this variety, well that leads us into the second area of your game you need to step up.

2. Increase your sources.

Start looking around locally for more consistent sources as well as looking into online sources.
Also start putting out ads, speaking to hunters and so on to increase your inconsistent sources.
Basically, I want you to increase the pool that you have to source your meats from so you can continue to seek out variety and just as importantly, have back up sources in case one falls through.

To wrap up, I want you to increase your dog's variety of foods, and increase the pool of sources you have to pull your food from.

Transitioning Puppies

In this section let's talk about transitioning puppies instead of adult dogs.

I told you I would teach you how to transition puppies, not just adult dogs and I meant it.
So don't worry and think you are going to have to read a whole separate book to figure out how to feed your puppy a raw diet.

The process is nearly identical. Some people may disagree with me and say that puppies need to be balanced from the start. I have nothing against balancing puppies from the start and if that's possible it is absolutely ideal. I would even go so far as to say that you should try to start puppies on a balanced diet from the start. However, if your puppy does not react to a balanced diet from the start certain steps should be taken. You can't just feed a puppy a balanced diet and ignore the fact that he or she is having diarrhea on a daily basis.

Puppies have the same potential for negative effects from the balanced from the start approach so I prefer to take them through the same slow transition as the adults.

At least I used to…

As we all grow and progress through our lives in our own respective fields we learn things, we're exposed to new information, and sometimes we change our opinions on certain topics. This is one of them. I am now an advocate of balancing puppies from the start when possible. However, if that does not go well then we need to go at this from a different angle.

I would rather a puppy not have a 100% perfectly balanced diet for a couple weeks than have to deal with issues like diarrhea if they aren't handling "balanced from the start" well. As you now know, dehydration can happen easily and can cause serious problems and death in extreme cases.

If you attempt to transition your puppy using a balanced from the start approach and they do not deal with it well, simplify things. Go back to just a white meat, bone in protein and only half the liver the calculator tells you that you need to feed on a daily basis. As soon as things are going well (holy grail poops) then slowly increase the liver and start adding non-liver organ after you reach 100% of the daily liver content. Once you reach 100% of your puppy's daily liver content, work on reaching 100% of your non-liver organ content.

Lastly, start adding in red meat slowly. After your puppy is successfully eating white meat, bone content, red meat, liver, and other organs, your puppy is transitioned.

If your puppy is having difficulty during any of these stages, it may be beneficial to look into supplements such as slippery elm bark and digestive supplements. As you should with any supplement, please read the directions carefully and research the supplement very well. I'll talk more about supplements in the next chapter.

How much do you feed puppies?

When it comes to puppies v.s adults there is simply a difference in feeding percentages and feeding frequency. The differences in feeding frequency and percentages is based on their age. Growing puppies need to be fed more often and need to be fed a higher percentage of their body weight.

I recommend that very young puppies under 12 months of age be fed 3 times a day. As they pass their 12 month mark twice a day feedings may be appropriate. For giant breed puppies it may be beneficial to extend that to 18 - 24 months.

Never do once a day feedings for puppies under 12-18 months of age.

It's also important to note that small breeds like chihuahuas may require a meat and bone ground mix to start with until they are a few months old and have the teeth and jaw strength to break down small meaty bone sources like wings.
We talked about that in the "Small dog considerations" section but I wanted to remind you.

Don't worry though, they'll get there.

The following percentages are based off the puppies **current** weight. As a simple math example if your puppy weighed 10 lbs then 10% would be 1 lb and so on.
It's important to note that these are not exact date or percentage amounts because you should be paying attention to your dog's weight and expected growth over time depending on their breed or mix of breed and their overall physique.

Meaning that dogs are individuals and if your dog is either super skinny or getting way too chubby then you need to modify these feeding percentages accordingly.

The time frames below dictate how much you should be feeding and at what age. Again, observe and adjust and consider dragging these percentage changes out if you have a giant breed puppy. (Great Dane and so on.)

- **Time Frame 1: 8 Weeks - 3/4 Months**
  - Feed 10% at the 8 week mark and end around 8% at the 3 to 4 month mark.
- **Time Frame 2: 3 Months - 6 Months**
  - Feed 8% at the 3-4 month mark and end around 6% at the 6 month mark.
- **Time Frame 3: 6 - 8 Months**

- Feed 6% at the 6 month mark and end around 4% at the 8 month mark.
- **Time Frame 4: 8 Months - 11 Months**
  - Feed 4% at the 8 month mark and end around 2-3 % at the 11 month mark.
- **12 - 18 Months**
  - Once you hit 12 months or 1 year old redo your calculations and start feeding your dog as an adult at 2% - 3% of their current body weight to maintain their weight as a starting point. If you have a giant breed puppy like a great dane, consider staying in the 3%-4% range of this final time frame.

Another important thing to remember is that growing puppies have greater calcium requirements than adult dogs. The frustrating part is that we don't really KNOW how much more!

To accomplish this consider feeding slightly higher than the recommended 10% of bone or supplementing calcium sources like egg shells into your puppy's diet. Don't go overboard though as too much calcium can cause issues.

There you have it, a simple to follow puppy transition guide.

Remember to feed the different percentages based on age and feed them more 2-3 times a day depending on their age, try to balance them from the start and if that doesn't work out back off a little bit and take things slow.

Side Note

Please research information regarding joint and cancer issues with puppies that are spayed or neutered too young. I know, way outside the scope of nutrition that this book is based off of but as someone with an adult dog suffering from joint issues because of this early I felt it deserved a few quick sentences.

Transitioning To B.A.R.F. Model Raw

In this section I want to talk about transitioning your dog to the raw B.A.R.F. diet. What to do first and what I think you should do when you make the switch.

So you've decided that you want to follow the B.A.R.F. model of raw feeding and want to include fruits and veggies in your dog's diet. That's AWESOME. I'm really excited for you. I do however have an opinion on what you should do first.

I've talked A LOT about going slow in this book, like a lot. Whether it's supplements, the initial switch to raw, adding new proteins, and so on. I don't think a transition to the B.A.R.F. model should be any different.

Now I'm not saying going straight from not feeding raw to feeding the B.A.R.F. model couldn't work, just like the slow transition v.s. Balanced from the start scenario, balanced from the start can work, I just don't think it has as high of a transition success rate with adult dogs.

At least not from my observations over the last several years.

With this in mind I suggest that you make the transition to prey model first using the transition methods in this chapter. Once you get the transition to prey model done, it's an easy step from A to B or prey model into B.A.R.F. model. Just get those fruits and veggies in and boom, you're feeding B.A.R.F..

When it comes to making that A to B transition I also have some suggestions.

Suggestion 1 - Don't drastically reduce meat content to make room for vegetables and fruit.

I believe that the B.A.R.F. model Kimberly Morris Gauthier feeds is ideal. She does not drastically reduce the meat content in her dogs' diets, she simply adds the fruits and veggies via a premade mix or now fermented vegetables.

That being said, some people DO temporarily reduce meat content and up veggie content during a weight loss period. Seek advice on that if you find yourself in that situation.

Suggestion 2 - Beware of starches & sugars.

Some vegetables are significantly higher in starches than others, or in fancy terms they have a high glycemic index. These starches are particularly bad for dogs with a tendency towards yeast issues so focus on feeding low starch vegetables like Kale. Check out Kimberly's veggie mix on keepthetailwagging.com for examples.

Fruits are always going to be high in sugars, it's why they are nature's candy. Please keep this in mind if you have a dog with diabetes or cancer. The sugars and carbohydrates are not good for dogs with either of those issues.

The bottomline here in my opinion is that I think you will have a much higher chance of a successful, issue free transition to the BARF diet if you implement the prey model diet first and then transition to the BARF diet.

Also, when you do make that transition don't drastically cut out meat to make room for the veggies and fruit, and keep the sugars and starches in the fruits and vegetables you add in mind when selecting what fruits and veggies you are going to feed.

Transitioning To Premade Raw

In this section I want to talk about transitioning your dog onto a pre-made raw diet.

It's probably the easiest transition there is but there are still a few key points I'd keep in mind so let's get right to them.

Like I said before, transitioning your dog onto a pre-made raw diet is probably the easiest way to do it. Why? Well because everything is right there for you. All you have to do is feed the patty or amount of the chub recommended by the company.

That being said there are a few points to consider when making this transition.

1. It's essentially a balanced from the start approach.

I talked earlier about the difference between slow transitions and balanced from the start transitions. I said that sometimes the balanced from the start transitions can be difficult on dogs because it's a lot of new things all at once. Keep this in mind when transitioning your dog to premade raw. There may be some runs or loose stools when you start.

2. Sometimes these premade raw products don't actually meet the 80/10/5/5 formula.

What I recommend is spend a week or two feeding the premade raw you decided on. During this 2-week period contact the company you chose to go with and ask them about the ratios of what is in the food. Some companies will put this on the packaging but you may still need to contact them for details. After this 2-week period of feeding just the premade raw product, start adding in anything that was missing from the premade raw.

For example, if the premade raw only included liver but no non-liver organs, start adding one.

3. Premade raw is expensive.

At first glance it's weird to think that people would go through the trouble of DIY models of raw feeding like prey model and BARF when you consider the fact that premade raw is readily available. Well it becomes overwhelmingly obvious when you start to look at the difference in cost.

Premade raw is **SIGNIFICANTLY** more expensive than the DIY models of raw feeding. Unless you have a small dog or an enormous budget, most people that start with premade raw eventually switch to a DIY model because they simply can't afford the premade for an extended period of time.

If you are in a situation where you really want to start with premade but know your finances can't maintain it long term, spend the time that you are feeding premade exploring DIY models.
Look for sources, re-read this chapter in the book, talk to other people that are feeding DIY models and so on. Basically, prepare yourself for the switch from premade to DIY.

4. Some companies recommend more food than necessary.

Sometimes you will see a premade raw product recommending a significantly larger amount of food per day than the calculator does. I don't know exactly why this is unless the premade has A LOT of vegetables and fruit and is lacking in calories so more needs to be fed.

If you follow the recommendations on a premade raw product and find that your dog is gaining weight while nothing else like activity levels have changed in their life, consider decreasing the amount of food you are feeding daily.

So there you have it, 4 points you should consider if you are going to switch your dog to a premade raw diet. It's a balanced from the start approach. Some premade products do not meet the 80/10/5/5 recommendations. Premade raw is much more expensive than DIY raw feeding models like prey model and BARF. Lastly, sometimes premade raw companies recommend what seems to be a much higher amount of food per day than the book's daily amount calculator recommends.

If you keep these things in mind you should have no trouble switching your dog over to a premade raw diet.

Introducing New Proteins After The Transition

In this section I want to cover something that every raw feeder has to figure out and that's how to integrate new proteins into the diet.

Let's get started.

Once you get through your initial transition you're going to want to start adding some variety to your dog's meals and by variety I mean new proteins from different animals.
Not only is this important for the overall quality of the diet, but believe it or not sometimes dogs get bored if they get the same thing all the time.

Now I'm not saying you need to be feeding 20 different proteins all the time in a constant rotation but you do need to provide a variety. Too many people I feel focus on this idea out there that you have to feed 50% white meat and 50% red meat.

Instead focus on variety. Feed as many different sources for white meat as you can and feed as many sources of red meat as you can and rotate them.

Typically, our dogs will get 2 different sets of meals for a two week period where we rotate back and forth between the two meals every other day. This keeps the dog's interested and their food sources varied. So how do you implement these new proteins into your dog's diet? I'll tell you.

You've heard me say this A LOT so further during this section and I'm going to say it again. START SLOW.

I full heartedly believe in slow approaches to everything when it comes to a dog's diet other than a few select, very urgent medical situations like a dog with cancer being put on a keto diet.

For more information on those types of situations check out thetruthaboutcancer.com or ketopetsanctuary.com, they have a free guide on ketogenic diets for dogs.

When you decide it's time to add a new protein to your dog's diet, start slow by adding maybe 10% to 25% of the total meat content for a particular meal, the same goes for organs.

Then you can slowly increase that amount as you look for any negative responses to that protein source that could indicate a possible allergy or intolerance.

If you happen to notice negative changes after implementing this new protein then you can easily remove it, see if the problem persists or subsides, and if it subsides, there is a possibility that your dog has an allergy to the new protein you tried to implement.

The main takeaways for this section are that variety is key and extremely important to the diet in regards to both overall diet quality AND your dog's satisfaction, and that you should start and implement new proteins slowly like you would a new supplement.

Start small and build up.

Chapter 8

General Information About Common Supplements

Common Supplements & If You Should Feed Them

This section of...sections, is going to be focused on supplements that you can add to your dog's diet. Notice and pay close attention to the fact that I said "can" and not "must" or "should". I wanted to take the time to make these sections just to give you an idea of what supplements are and when you should consider feeding them. Just as, if not more importantly. I want to tell you when NOT to feed a supplement.

Unless of course you want to end up like my raw feeding BFF Kimberly Gauthier who in her early years of raw feeding, ended up with what she described as a "mad scientist's lab" in her kitchen comprised of one supplement for her dogs after the other.

Let's get to it.

What is a supplement?

A supplement is something that is formulated to address a specific need, relieve a particular issue, and so on. In fact by definition a supplement is "something that completes or enhances something else when added to it."

I like to think of it this way. When the needs of our dogs are not being fully met or fulfilled by a raw diet alone, supplementation can help us complete or enhance the raw diet that we are feeding. So by supplementing a raw food diet, we are completing or enhancing what a raw food diet is already doing for our dogs.

SO, we should feed every supplement that we can get our hands on and that we can afford right? *Ehhh! Wrong.

In my humble opinion we should be thinking about supplementation exactly in the way that it is defined, as something we use to complete or enhance our dog's diets and lives. In other words, using supplementation to address specific problems, fulfill particular needs, or enhance health.

So if our dog is starting to have joint issues then we can use a glucosamine or other joint supplement to complete and meet our dog's needs. Turmeric paste is what I use for my dog's joint issues that stem both from his breed and the early neutering his original owner had done.

If we own a breed that is known for particular issues like joint problems that are worsened by inflammation we can supplement with an all-natural supplement like turmeric paste.

The point is that we should be using supplements to meet our dog's needs and fill the gaps in their nutritional health that are not being met by their diet alone, not just because a label tells us it's a wonder supplement.

When should you NOT feed a supplement?

Knowing when not to feed a supplement really boils down to 1 phrase, "Just because."
If you are considering feeding a supplement "Just because" a friend said that it's awesome, or "Just because" someone on the internet said you should, you probably shouldn't.

When it comes down to whether or not you should be providing a supplement to your dog ask yourself these questions.

Question 1 - Was this recommended by a veterinarian, preferably a holistic vet?

If your vet has been working with you on resolving a specific issue then their opinion shouldn't be discounted without very good reason such as the opinion of a second veterinarian.

Question 2 - What hole in your dog's diet are you trying to fill?

If you can't identify the exact hole in the diet that the supplement you are considering is going to fill, then you probably don't need to be feeding that supplement.

Question 3 - What problem or issue am I trying to solve or address?

If you can't identify the exact problem or issue that you are considering feeding a supplement for, then you probably don't need to be feeding that supplement.

Question 4 - Does this supplement have a proven track record?

Is there any actual evidence, even if it's just well documented via social media / anecdotal proof that this supplement solves the problem you're trying to address?

Question 5 - Is the supplement being provided by a company you can trust?

If that supplement does have a proven track record, is it being provided by a company that has a reputation for quality? The best way to find this out is to see if the company has third party testing, if they have a lot of great reviews from previous customers, and if they are willing to speak with you in detail about questions you have about the product.

One more thing to consider when it comes to supplementation is that you should start slow. Don't read the label and give a full dose the first time around. Start with ¼ of the recommended amount or possibly less if ¼ still seems to be a lot and work your way up to a full dose slowly.
This is especially important for dogs that have a history of being sensitive to changes in their diet.

All in all supplements can be an absolutely amazing addition when it comes to providing proper nutrition and health. Just keep in mind that you should never feed or provide a supplement "Just because" and make sure that you ARE feeding a supplement to complete or enhance your dog's overall diet and health.

Feeding Coconut Oil

Unless you've been living under a rock for the last 5 years you've probably seen and heard a lot of things about coconut oil so let's take a look at what it is and how it can benefit your dog.

What is Coconut Oil and where does it come from?

Coconut oil is an oil that is extracted from the meat of mature coconuts. The meat is that white part on the inside of the coconut. Coconut oil also contains medium chain triglyceride or MCTs, I'll talk about why that's important in just a moment.

What are the benefits of Coconut Oil?

The benefits of coconut oil and/or MCTs are many, here's a few of them.

#1 MCTs are what you could call an extremely powerful "brain food".

A study consisting of 24 beagles showed that after 1 month of MCTs being supplemented in their diets they showed drastic improvements in cognitive abilities including the ability to learn. It's even believed that sources of MCTs like coconut oil could slow down cognitive degeneration in aging dogs. That way you CAN teach old dogs new tricks. I know, I know, another lame joke. Moving on.

#2 Coconut can help with weight loss.

MCTs cannot be stored as fat and even provide a feeling of being satiated, coconut oil can be a great advantage in helping your dog lose a few pounds.

#3 Coconut oil is anti-everything it would seem.

Coconut oil has been shown to be anti-fungal, anti-viral, and anti-microbial so not only is it great for the dog to digest but it can be used topically for some minor cuts and abrasions.

#4 Coconut oil also provides a lot of support for healthy skin and a shiny coat.

#5 MCTs help transport omega 3 fatty acids throughout the body.

A lot of people feed some type of omega 3 fatty acid supplement like fish or krill oil and these supplements become even more effective when combined with the transportation support of MCTs that are found in the coconut oil.

I could go on and on with the benefits of coconut oil and MCTs but these are a few of the big ones. I encourage you to do some more research to dive even deeper on this supplement.

What dogs could benefit from Coconut Oil?

Given the list of benefits I just listed, consider feeding coconut oil to dogs that
have a high amount of cognitive demand like SAR dogs or dogs that compete in some type of skill based sport, dogs that could stand to lose a few pounds, dogs that are getting into their later years, dogs being fed some type of omega 3 fatty acid supplement or whole fish for omega-3s, and dogs with dry skin and dull coats.

Feeding Tips

Like anything else I recommend starting slow with coconut oil as it can cause an upset stomach if the dog is not used to it. Not only can you just feed it straight from the jar, you can also mix it with other foods like liver and an egg if you are having trouble getting your dog to eat liver or other organ.

Another great use for coconut oil is to use it in conjunction with turmeric and a few other ingredients to make what is called golden paste or turmeric paste. They're the same thing. If you don't want to deal with the mess of coconut oil, there are powdered versions of coconut "oil" and MCTs available on the market.

Feeding Fish Oil

I don't think that I could name many, if any other supplement that is as widely used and talked about as fish oil. Let's dive right into the fishy waters that is fish oil...I have GOT to stop making these stupid jokes.

What is fish oil and where does it come from?

Fish oil is made from cold water fish like herring, salmon, and mackerel. The fish is then put through a process that separates the oil from the rest of the fish and boom you have fish oil. There are a lot more steps to the process but that's the beginning and end of what happens.

Fish oil is one of the most commonly supplemented sources of Omega-3 fatty acids that we have available to us. Omega-3's are so important in a dog's diet because it's impossible for the dog's body to produce Omega-3's on it's own.

There are 3 main types of Omega-3 fatty acids.

EPA & DHA - The 1st & 2nd Omega-3 Fatty Acids

These are typically found in the same sources, in other words, where you find EPA you'll typically find DHA. EPA & DHA are found in lots of sea creatures like fish, squid, krill, and even phytoplankton.

ALA - The 3rd Omega-3 Fatty Acid

ALA is typically found in the oil of plants like hemp and flax seeds. Unfortunately, ALA has to be converted into EPA & DHA before the dog's body can use it. EPA & DHA are superior sources of Omega-3 fatty acids because there are no additional steps that the dog's body has to go through to utilize the Omega-3's like there would be if the Omega-3 source had been ALA.

What are the benefits of fish oil?

When all is said and done the list of benefits for fish oil / omega-3 fatty acids is at the very least extensive.

- Omega 3- fatty acids have anti-inflammatory properties

- They help with joint point problems.
- Improve coat quality.
- Supports healthy skin by helping prevent itching, scratching, and chewing.
- Omega 3 fatty acids help dogs live longer lives
- Improves a dog's ability to learn and overall memory. (In other words it's brain fuel which makes teaching spot how to sit that much easier.)
- They improve cardiovascular health.
- The list goes on...

What dogs could benefit from fish oil?

Saying what dogs could benefit from omega 3 fatty acids or fish oil is an easy one, all of them. Like I said earlier omega-3 fatty acids are a necessary part of a dog's diet and the dog's body cannot produce them on it's own. With cold water fish like mackerel and herring having some of highest levels of EPA & DHA, it's easy to see why fish oil is such a popular choice & source for omega-3 fatty acids.

That being said, there are lots of alternatives out there for omega 3 fatty acids that you can look into like krill oil and phytoplankton that I mentioned earlier in the section. This is important as there is more and more evidence coming out regarding concerns about fish oil like oxidation and the oil going rancid after it's opened.

Feeding Tips

Depending on whether you choose fish oil or some other type Omega 3 supplement, the dosage is going to vary greatly.

Always read your labels before starting a regimen of fish oil or any other Omega-3 supplement and remember to start slow. Somewhere around ¼ the recommended dosage is what I generally recommend. You can then increase that amount until you reach the full dosage over a couple weeks.

ONE FINAL NOTE

Whatever source of omega-3 you decide on, fish oil, krill oil, phytoplankton, or fresh food sources you MUST provide omega-3 in one way or another. It is an absolutely essential ingredient to a healthy, balanced raw food diet.

Feeding Turmeric

What is turmeric and where does it come from?

Turmeric comes from the turmeric root. Turmeric is part of the ginger family which isn't surprising when you put the 2 roots side by side. Turmeric contains a compound that is called curcumin. Curcumin is the active ingredient in turmeric and is what makes turmeric such a powerful supplement.

What are the benefits of turmeric?

- Antioxidant
- Anti-inflammatory
- Antibacterial
- Help some dogs with diarrhea
- Thins the blood and reduces the chance of blood clots.
- Reduces allergy symptoms
- Promotes healthy digestion.

When you consider this long list of benefits it's not hard to guess why turmeric has been labeled as another wonder or superfood.

What dogs could benefit from turmeric?

Turmeric, when implemented properly can be an asset in just about any dog's diet. That being said, you need to remember the blood thinning properties that turmeric possesses. So if you have a dog that is on blood thinning medications turmeric may not be for that dog.

If you do have a dog on blood thinning medications, it's important to speak with a holistic veterinarian before adding turmeric to your dog's supplement rotation.

Feeding Tips

Turmeric powder is available and can be fed on it's own but turmeric paste or golden paste as some call it is significantly more effective at delivering the benefits that turmeric has to offer. Additionally, it's easier to hide in that form if your dog doesn't like the flavor. I hide it in organs and feed it before anything else. Doing it this way also prevents the dog from getting the turmeric paste all over the place which can cause TERRIBLE stains.

Here's an easy recipe you can follow. You're going to need:

- 1 ½ cups of fresh water (alkaline or filtered if possible)
- ½ cup of turmeric powder (organic if possible)
- ⅓ cup of coconut oil (organic if possible)
- 1 - 1 ½ teaspoons of freshly ground pepper (the fresh ground part is important)

Step 1

Add the water and turmeric powder into a pot, stir well and let it simmer for 7-10 minutes until it thickens and turns into a paste. If it dries up before it turns into a paste you can add more water.

Step 2

Once the water and powder turn into paste, add the coconut oil while the paste is still warm and mix well. A whisk works best for this but just about anything will do the trick.

Step 3

After your coconut oil is mixed into the paste well add your pepper and mix it all up again.

Step 4

You can then put it in a glass jar in the fridge for a couple of weeks or freeze it for later use.

Like any other supplement it's important to start with small amounts and slowly let the dog's body adjust to the recommended dosage. Starting with ¼ teaspoon is plenty. It's recommended that you feed up to ¼ tsp per 10 lbs of body weight but many have found that as little s ½ tsp a day is a sufficient amount to reap the benefits of turmeric paste. If I feed my dog any more than ½ tsp every other day it starts to upset hit stomach. If you start to see the runs, you've gone past a good amount for your dog. Back it off a little but until things settle down and then you've found a good daily amount for your dog.

It's important to note that you do not need to feed it every day to reap the benefits. Like I just mentioned, I only provide it every other day and my dog is still benefiting from it.

Pro Tip

When you are preparing turmeric or golden paste use utensils and containers that do not stain easily and wear gloves if you don't want to have orange hands for a week. Turmeric stains very easily so i also wouldn't recommend wearing your favorite shirt while you prepare turmeric paste.

Feeding Slippery Elm Bark

If you've ever seen a post in a raw feeding Facebook group where the poster is asking for suggestions on relieving the runs or loose stools, then almost without a doubt you've seen someone recommend slippery elm bark.

What is slippery elm bark and where does it come from?

Slippery Elm or Slippery Elm Bark as it is sometimes called comes from the stringy inner bark of the slippery elm tree.

What are the benefits of slippery elm bark?

In the simplest terms slippery elm lubricates and relieves inflammation inside the body.
Because of this it is able to solve a wide variety of problems including coughing, diarrhea, and constipation. It's weird to think that one supplement will help diarrhea and constipation but if we look at what slippery elm does it makes perfect sense.

Oftentimes, diarrhea is caused by some type of irritation in the body that in turn causes inflammation. By reducing the inflammation and lubricating the lining of the digestive tract, you are helping the body prevent more irritation that could be causing the diarrhea.

When it comes to constipation it makes just as much sense. If your dog is "backed up" and just can't get a movement to pass, reducing inflammation and swelling in the digestive tract while also lubricating the tract with the slippery elm bark can go a long way toward helping "move things along".

What dogs could benefit from slippery elm bark?

If your dog has been suffering from a cough or is experiencing diarrhea or constipation then slippery elm may be what you're looking for. It wouldn't hurt just to keep some around to have on hand just in case.

Feeding Tips

Like many supplements slippery elm or slippery elm bark comes in a variety of forms. Pills, powders, and so on. It's important to read the labels and dosing instructions on the labels of these different supplements.

Feeding Colostrum

What is colostrum and where does it come from?

Colostrum is a liquid that mammals produce (yes even humans) typically just before and after birth. Colostrum's biological purpose is to provide the infant with things that it needs to protect itself against disease. Antibodies and elevated levels of fat and protein help do this.

What are the benefits of colostrum?

Aside from the being extremely beneficial for infants, colostrum is known for a wide range of benefits. Some of these benefits include helping with leaky gut which can cause issues like yeast, supporting the bodies fight against cancer by producing white blood cells that attack cancer, and many more.

Undoubtedly one of the largest talked about benefits of colostrum is it's ability to help the body manage allergies. Colostrum can help regulate an overactive immune system, or kick an immune system lacking activity into overdrive.

Colostrum like I mentioned earlier also indirectly helps with allergies by helping alleviate leaky gut syndrome which is a major contributor to allergies overall in the dog's body.

What dogs could benefit from colostrum?

If your dog experiences seasonal allergies, leaky gut syndrome, yeast issues, or some type of allergy like environmental allergies, it may be worth looking deeper into colostrum and eventually supplementing your dog's diet with it.

Feeding Tips

Colostrum can be provided to your dog in a variety of ways. Colostrum can come in pill form, powder form, or in it's raw liquid form. Some argue that the raw form that is often sold in glass bottles is significantly more potent but others claim they experience benefits that are just as effective from the other alternatives.

Each type of colostrum source (pill, powder, or raw liquid) have different feeding instructions. It's important to do your research when deciding to implement colostrum as a supplement to ensure you are providing the proper amounts.

Feeding Kefir

What is kefir and where does it come from?

Kefir is made from kefir grains and goat, sheep, or cow's milk. The best part is the grains can be used more than once. Kefir is also often referred to as milk kefir because you are adding kefir grains and some type of milk together.

For a great recipe for DIY Kefir, go to keepthetailwagging.com and search the term "DIY Milk Kefir for Dogs". It's easier than you'd think.

What are the benefits of kefir?

- Kefir boosts the immune system
- Absolutely destroys yeast
- Helps gassy dogs
- Natural probiotic
- Helps fight allergies
- Supports healthy digestion

What dogs could benefit from kefir?

Unless your dog has an extreme lactose issue then just about any dog would be a good candidate for kefir being added to the diet. Yeasty dogs, gassy dogs, and dogs with allergies are some of the dogs that could really benefit from kefir being added to their diets.

Feeding Tips

Kefir is powerful stuff, because of this it doesn't take more than a few tablespoons a few days a week for your dog to reap all the benefits of being fed kefir.

Feeding Raw Goat's Milk

What is raw goat's milk and where does it come from?

Surprise surprise, raw goat's milk come from...goats. Weird right? With it being RAW goat's milk, this means that it is of course unpasteurized. You can buy raw goat's milk from some online raw food suppliers as well as local pet stores and farmers markets.

What are the benefits of raw goat's milk?

Raw goat's milk is a widely used supplement because of it's ability to help with a lot of chronic and non-chronic diseases and issues.

Some of the benefits of goat's milk:
- Helps with liver disease.
- Helps with kidney stones and chronic kidney disease.
- It digests very quickly.
- Helps with poor digestion.
- Helps with diabetes.
- And can even help dogs with diarrhea.

What dogs could benefit from raw goat's milk?

Well first off, raw goat's milk could be a great thing for almost any dog purely because it supports proper digestion. Beyond that, any dog that suffers from chronic liver or kidney disease, kidney stones, poor digestion or sporadic bouts of diarrhea would all be great candidates for raw goat's milk supplementation.

Feeding Tips

Some people concern themselves over the lactose in raw goat's milk claiming that their dogs are lactose intolerant which may or may not be true.

What I can tell you is that raw goat's milk has significantly lower levels of lactose than traditional milk that comes from cows. If you decide that raw goat's milk is for you, feeding a few ounces of raw goat's milk a few days a week is going to be great for your dog. Never feed too much at once and like anything else start slow if your dog has never had it before.

Feeding Enzymes, Prebiotics, & Probiotics

In this section I want to talk about Digestive Enzymes, Probiotics, and Prebiotics. All three of these things are extremely important when it comes to your dog's health because they support the gut. It's been said more than once that a healthy gut equals a healthy dog. Let's get started.

First let's look at these 3 things and what they do for your dog.

Digestive Enzymes

Digestive enzymes perform the duty of breaking down food so it can be digested and absorbed. We once thought that feeding green tripe alone was enough to cover digestive enzymes in the diet. While it's true that green tripe comes with a long list of benefits including digestive enzymes, there just isn't enough to do the job on it's own.

Probiotics

Probiotics are often referred to as "good" bacteria in your dog's gut. Your dog's body cannot create probiotics on it's own especially in dogs with chronic issues like allergies and digestive upset.

Keep probiotics in mind when a dog suddenly start having issues like diarrhea. This is important because it could be a sign that your dog's gut is lacking a sufficient amount of good bacteria. By adding a probiotic to your dog's diet, you can get things back in order by renewing the amount of good bacteria in your dog's gut.

Prebiotics

Prebiotics are just as important as digestive enzymes and probiotics. Particularly because prebiotics help feed and grow the good bacteria or probiotics in your dog's gut. It was once thought that prebiotics did more bad than good because it was assumed that they were also feeding and growing the bad bacteria.

Luckily this has been proven to not be true and the only thing that the prebiotics are supporting is the good bacteria.

The main benefit of these 3 powerhouse supplements is that they provide your dog with a healthy, well functioning gut. So if your dog has chronic digestive issues like diarrhea, bad gas, immune issues or chronic ear infections, these 3 powerhouses may be worth looking into.

Feeding Tips

With the wide range of types these supplements come in like powders, pills, and paste it would be impossible for me to accurately recommend a proper amount or dosage for these supplements.

Make sure that you do more in depth research about the product you want to supplement and pay close attention to dosage recommendations from the manufacturer. If you do decide to feed these supplements make sure that you are using a high quality product from a reputable resource that is manufacturing them with dogs in mind.

Feeding Glucosamine

What is glucosamine and where does it come from?

Glucosamine can either be synthetically created or sourced from natural materials.
Glucosamine is actually a combination of 2 things. Glucose which is a sugar, and glutamine which is an amino acid. Glucosamine works with other things in your body to help build cartilage. It occurs naturally in the body but as dogs age glucosamine production is

reduced which is why older dogs sometimes start to show signs of joint issues. This makes providing glucosamine to your dog super important especially if you have an older dog.

What are the benefits of glucosamine?

Glucosamine provides your dog's body with a lot of benefits.

- Like I already mentioned it plays a key role in building cartilage in your dog's joints.
- Glucosamine is also anti-inflammatory.
- Glucosamine is also critical in reducing arthritis pain in and improving movement in aging dogs.
- Glucosamine as a supplement helps fill the gap left by the reduction in natural glucosamine production as your dog ages.

What dogs could benefit from glucosamine?

- Dogs with arthritis.
- Dogs with hip or elbow dysplasia.
- Aging or senior dogs.

Feeding Tips

Like I mentioned earlier, glucosamine can be derived from either natural sources or synthetic sources. It's important that whenever possible you choose natural sources. Now I'm not saying synthetic sources are bad but you the body will recognize and better utilize natural sources which means that you are going to have to provide less than you would if you were using a synthetic source.

If you really want to dive deep look into receptors being clogged by synthetic glucosamine sources. But that's definitely not 101 stuff so save it for later after you are through the initial transition.

If you are going to go with synthetic sources for glucosamine pay close attention to the dosage recommendations on the label.

When it comes to natural sources just make sure you are providing a variety of high cartilage sources like bones with cartilage on them, duck and chicken feet, trachea, and knuckle bones.

Feeding Honey

What is honey and where does it come from?

Once again it is pretty obvious to tell where this supplement / food comes from. It's important whenever possible to get locally sourced honey, more on that in a moment.

What are the benefits of honey?

- Honey is full of natural enzymes
- Supports healthy digestion
- Is slowly released throughout the body so it is a great source of natural, long term energy.
- Is anti-bacterial, anti-microbial, anti-fungal, anti-inflammatory
- Is packed full of antioxidants...geez this is a lot of antis...
- & provides allergy relief. Here's where the sourcing locally comes in.

Because bees are using the natural pollens around them to make their honey, it's believed that dogs with environmental allergies will be able to slowly build up a tolerance for these allergens through the micro exposure to the pollens found in the honey.

Think of it as a natural vaccine on a much smaller scale. You are introducing the thing that could cause the body harm in small amounts giving the body a chance to build up a tolerance or defense against that particular thing.

What dogs could benefit from honey?

If you have a dog that suffers from environmental allergies, has consistent digestive issues, or has an extremely active lifestyle you may want to consider adding honey into your dog's diet.

Feeding Tips

I recommend that you always do your own research when it comes to dosage and feeding amounts, there is a general amount of honey that is often recommended. Approximately 1 tablespoon per day for large dogs and one teaspoon for small dogs.

Again, do your own research because science figures out new things everyday and these are just general guidelines.

I'll leave you with one cautionary statement.

If you have a dog with diabetes or cancer please consult a holistic vet before feeding honey. This is because the sugars in honey could be doing more harm than good in some cases.

Chapter 9

Additional Information

Activity Based Feeding Modifications

In this section I want to talk about a super important, but often overlooked topic and that is changing the amount of food you are feeding your dog based on changes in their activity levels. It doesn't have to be complicated but it does need to be done. Let's get started.

In the raw feeding world we're constantly seeing people give advice on how much to feed to maintain weight, gain weight, lose weight, etc…

With all this talk about maintaining, gaining, and losing weight, you would think that activity levels would end up in the middle of each of those conversations. Unfortunately, it doesn't happen very often and when it does happen it's fairly quickly overlooked and treated as an afterthought.

This isn't necessarily anyone's fault because we get so fixated on the percentages that are based off the dog's current weight and so on. I can tell you though from first hand experience that activity levels and modifying the amount of food you are feeding based on changes in activity levels can have a major impact on your dog's weight and therefore overall health.

A few summer's this book was written, my oldest dog Wolken somehow ended up burning the pads on all 4 of his feet. To this day I still don't know how it happened. At the time I was doing a lot of barefoot walking and tested the surfaces with my own feet, tested the asphalt with the back of my hand and everything seemed fine but however it happened, it happened.

Wolken's activity levels went down significantly for a few weeks as I'm sure you can imagine and we could no longer walk him on the asphalt, again for obvious reasons.

So here we have a case where a dog's activity levels dropped drastically and immediately. Additionally, I made ZERO changes to the amount of food he was eating. Can you guess what happened? Yup, Wolken gained a bunch of weight.

At the time it didn't even cross my mind to alter his feeding amounts because he had been eating the same amount for so long and prep time was basically an auto pilot experience.

One day I looked at Wolken and literally said out loud, "You're gettin' a little chubby buddy."

Long story short...well I guess it's too late for that...but anyways…long story short I reevaluated his weight, reduced the amount of food that I was feeding him, increased his activity levels slowly over time so he didn't become overwhelmed or injured and the weight started melting off.

These days he is or is very close to a healthy pet weight as my friend Ronny LeJeune would say. He moves well, doesn't look like a bag of jelly when he runs, has a nice "tucked waist", and is showing the slightest hint of his last few ribs. Wolken is ready for bikini season.

So how can YOU make sure you are properly adjusting feeding amounts when your dog's activity levels change?

Well there are 2 main ways. You can either reactively change the feeding percentage, or you can proactively change the feeding percentages. Let's take a look at what both of these methods look like.

Reactively changing your dog's feeding percentages:

Reactively is really the inferior way to do it between the 2 options. That being said, a minor increase or decrease in activity can compound in weight gain or loss overtime. So sometimes observing a change in your dog and then reacting to it is the only way to do it without exceptional time and effort. My "You're gettin' a little chubby buddy." was the beginning of my reactive change in Wolken's feeding percentages and overall health regimen. I.E. modified feeding percentages AND increased activity and play time.

You observe either weight gain or weight loss and change your feeding percentages accordingly. The problem with this method is that obviously the damage is already done. Your dog has already gained or lost a bunch of weight and now you have to correct it.

Proactively changing your dog's feeding percentages:

Out of the two ways this is definitely the superior method. When you proactively change your dog's diet you are being aware of the fact that your dog's activity levels are changing and you are going to change your feeding percentages accordingly.

An example would be a dog that just got signed up to train in ring work or some other high energy output sport and you know they are going to be burning a significantly higher amount of calories and overall energy. More is being put out so more needs to go in.

The benefit of this method is you are making changes in the feeding percentages BEFORE the weight is gained or lost so there is less work for you and your dog to do to keep them at a healthy weight

Goooo Slooow

When you are modifying these feeding percentages (hopefully in a proactive way) do it little bits at a time. Whether you are going up in feeding percentages or down in percentages start with .5%.

In other words, if your dog just started a new high energy sport and you are currently feeding 2.5%, try bumping it up to 3%. On the other side of the coin, if your dog is going to have a significant decrease in activity for one reason or another and you are feeding 2.5% consider dropping it to 2%. If this drop in activity is because of a major surgery then I encourage you to work with your veterinarian before significantly decreasing feeding percentages.

Whether you are trying to increase or decrease the amount of food you are feeding, change it slowly and continue feeding more or less by gauging your dog's weight gain or loss.

If you feed too little, you could be depriving your dog's body of necessary nutrients and fuel.

If you feed too much, especially if your dog is starting a new sport, you are asking for all kinds of problems by increasing your feeding percentages too much and causing rapid weight gain.

The name of this whole "modifying feeding percentages based on activity levels" game is all about awareness and observation.

Remember…"Observe & Adjust".

Feeding Bone Broth

In this additional information section, I want to take about bone broth. You've probably seen or heard about bone broth a lot over the last couple of years both for humans and dogs.

Let's take a look at what bone broth is, why people feed, whether or not it's really safe, and a loose recipe on how to make it.

What Is Bone Broth?

Bone broth can be extremely simple to make as far as steps and ingredients go but can be more complex depending on what you choose to add to it. Some people only add bones to their bone broth while some people get more complex by adding things like garlic, raw apple cider vinegar, healthy veggies like kale and broccoli and so on.

To put it in the simplest terms possible, bone broth is the after product of placing bones in water, slow cooking it for a long period of time that sometimes has other ingredients added to it and is extremely beneficial for dogs.

Why do people feed it?

Bone broth has quite the list of benefits that makes it a no brainer to figure out why people feed it.

- Bone broth can be added to kibble diets to give a boost of nutrients and moisture to the dog's diet. The moisture is particularly helpful since kibble requires so much more moisture to digest than raw foods.
- Bone broth is easy to digest and easy on an upset stomach which makes it perfect for getting some nutrients into dogs that are sick and are having a hard time keeping solid foods down.
- Bone broth can be very enticing for dogs that don't have an appetite for whatever reason which can be really important if sickness has caused the appetite loss.
- Bone broth is extremely nutritious and can be even more nutritious depending on what you add to it besides the bones.

- Bone broth is great for supporting joint health.
- Bone broth can be frozen for later use so you can do large batches of it and have homemade bone broth for a very long time without having to constantly restock/make your supply.

Is it safe for dogs to eat?

There have been some concerns circulating around the internet over the years about the dangers of feeding bone broth. These concerns are mainly focused on lead and glutamic acid.

The concerns are that the animals we feed are being exposed to higher amounts of lead which ends up in the bones we use for bone broth and that too much bone broth can cause neurological issues because of over exposure to an amino acid called glutamic acid.

The problem with citing these issues as "dangers" is that you would have to feed a very large amount of bone broth on a consistent basis before these started being a real concern.

If you can simply limit your bone broth feeding to necessary situations and or only feeding for supplementation purposes one to a few times a week you will easily avoid these "dangers" of feeding bone broth.

So how do you make it?

I don't know lol All joking aside it's unlikely your bone broth will be identical to anyone else's depending on how much of what you add to it but here is a simple recipe that you can add to overtime as you gain more experience.

Step 1

Pull out a slow cooker or crock pot of some kind.

Step 2

Add as many bones as you can while leaving room for an inch or two of water above the bones. Make sure to include plenty of bone sources that have a lot of joints like duck and chicken feet. These add a big boost to the joint benefits for your dog. Other bones you could add would include ribs, marrow bones, and shoulder bones.

Step 3

At this point you can add in a heaping spoonful of fresh garlic. If you are doing it with whole garlic, a few diced cloves will do. If you haven't heard of all the amazing benefits of garlic, do some googling. In large amounts it can be toxic for dogs but in smaller amounts it has several benefits.

Don't believe all the negativity surrounding it. Do the research and come to an educated conclusion on your own. If you're not comfortable with that it's okay, garlic isn't required to feel free to skip this step.

Step 4

Fill the pot with water, remember to not only cover the bones but fill it an inch or so above the bones. You want everything covered.

Step 5

Add a few teaspoons of raw apple cider vinegar, organic if possible. Don't go crazy on being exact with this, it will work out if you add a little extra.

Step 6

Turn your slow cooker on high for a few hours (I do it for about 2 hours) and then turn it to low. Cook it for 24 - 48 hours. I usually end up somewhere in the middle. After several hours have passed and it has reached a good temperature, stir the broth regularly from that point forward.

Step 7

Turn off the slow cooker and remove all bones and meat left over in the slow cooker. Feed the meat as a treat or freeze for later and toss the bones. Store your bone broth in containers like glass mason jars or freeze it into ice cubes.

IMPORTANT NOTE

Never ever feed your dog a cooked bone. Make sure you dispose of the cooked bones in a place where your dog cannot get to them. Preferably in the outside trash can.

You're all done! Have fun with bone broth, look up other people's recipes, experiment, and remember to not feed it too often and you'll be an "expert" in no time.

Calcium & Phosphorus

This particular section will cover a topic that is biologically significant but often just confuses and overwhelms new feeders. Unnecessarily in my opinion. Don't get me wrong, it's an important subject but sometimes I feel that it is overblown in online raw feeding communities.

For that reason, this section is one of the sections in the "additional information" chapter as I do not feel it is necessary to know in order to start the diet.

With that in mind this will be a very simple explanation of the concept of balancing calcium and phosphorus in your dog's diet. If you are an information junkie and really want to delve deep into the science on this one I highly recommend you search the web to satisfy your curiosity. Be ready for some brain pain though.

What Is Calcium?

It's difficult to say exactly what calcium is used for without going into the scientific explanations I was trying to avoid in this book that is geared towards beginners. So for now, I'll just say that calcium is important for cell integrity, immune health, skeletal health and more. Dog's need lots calcium and puppies need even more like I referenced in chapter 7.

For these reasons, it is critical that you don't let your fear of whole bones or bone in grinds scare you into feeding a boneless diet. It's simply not healthy or balanced and will lead to a plethora of issues. Bones are high in both calcium and phosphorus which is why they are SO CRUCIAL to a raw diet. A boneless diet is ESPECIALLY damaging if you do it with puppies who are using A LOT of calcium during their first stages of life.

What Is Phosphorus?

Phosphorus's primary responsibility (but certainly not only responsibility) is to assist in the growth of teeth and bones throughout the body. Phosphorus can be found in very high amounts in muscle meat, muscle meat also happens to be very low in calcium.

So what does all of this mean and how to you balance these things?

Well what it really means is that calcium and phosphorus play key roles in the body on multiple levels and imbalances can cause lots of problems. The good news is that it is, for the most part, exceptionally difficult to cause deficiencies with calcium and phosphorus unless you are feeding an extremely unbalanced diet like a diet with no bones or a diet with WAAAY too much bone.

If you are following a raw diet with approximately 80% muscle meat and approximately 10% bone, maybe slightly more bone depending on your dog (and definitely more if you are feeding a puppy) then you are coming really close to balancing calcium phosphorus.

In other words, feed your dog a raw diet, follow the "secret formula" I discussed in an earlier chapter and you will be okay.

Again though, if you are a science nerd and really want to get to the bottom of this I recommend you dig around, read books, and continue your learning.

The book "Canine Nutrigenomics by W. Jean Dodds - DVM, & Diana R. Laverdure is an excellent place to start."

Chapter 10

So You're Feeding Raw...What Now?

What Now?

Congratulations!!

You are feeding raw, are about to start, or you are well your way. So what do you do now? I'll tell you exactly what to do RIGHT NOW.

Right now, as you read this book, make me, your dog or dogs, any future dogs you may have, and most importantly yourself ONE promise.

Just one.

Promise that you will never stop learning and that you will always be open to new information about raw feeding as it comes out.

New studies are happening **RIGHT NOW** and will continue to happen as more of the world is made aware of this amazing "new" way to feed our furry best friends and family members. As these studies come out some of current beliefs about raw feeding and the best way to do things may be challenged. As you now know, I experienced this first hand in regards to whether or not vegetables have a place in the canine diet.

We can't **ever** let that feeling of being challenged or our egos get in the way of learning and doing the absolute best we can for our dogs.

So please, right now, make that promise. Actually read this out loud!

Right here and right now….

…I promise to never stop learning about raw feeding and fresh foods for my pets...

…and I promise I will always keep my mind open to new information…

…even if that new information challenges my current beliefs…

…my ego and beliefs are not important…

…my dog's health…

…my dog's quality of life…

…and the amount of time I get to spend with my furry family members are what really counts…

…I promise I will never let my ego or beliefs come before my dog's health.

Thank you so much for purchasing this book, supporting my mission to bring raw feeding to more dog owners, and for taking the time to do the very best you can for your dog or dogs.

I'm Scott Jay Marshall II, "Dog Dad" of RawFeeding101.com and...

Remember, you don't have to be perfect to be an amazing dog owner. You just have to do your best every day and try to improve as you go forward.

Peace. :)

Online & Recommended Resources

Raw Feeding 101 Downloadable Resources

Visit the link below to download the Raw Feeding 101 daily amount calculators.

www.rawfeeding101.com/calculators

This includes:
- Raw Feeding 101 Daily Amount Calculator (pounds & ounces version)
- Raw Feeding 101 Daily Amount Calculator (grams & kilograms version)
- Bone Content Calculator

Recommended Raw Feeding Resources

People to follow on social media:
- Kimberly Morris Gauthier
- Ronny LeJeune
- Rodney Habib
- Dr. Karen Becker
- Gregori Lukas
- Kohl Harrington

Websites:
- www.dogdadofficial.com
- www.rawfeeding101.com
- www.keepthetailwagging.com
- www.perfectlyrawsome.com
- www.therawfeedingcommunity.com
- www.petfooled.com
- www.dogcancerseries.com
- www.dogsnaturallymagazine.com
- www.longlivingpets.com

Books:
- A Novice's Guide to Raw Feeding for Dogs
- Canine Nutrigenomics
- Raw Feeding Meal Tracking Journal
- Raw and Thriving
- Dr. Becker's Real Food For Healthy Dogs and Cats

Facebook Groups:
- Raw Feeding 101 - Learn To Feed Raw
- Raw Feeding University (RFU)
- The Raw Feeding Community

Other:
- The Raw Feeding Breakfast Bowl (Facebook & YouTube)
- Pet Fooled (Netflix)
- Long Living Pets
  - Ongoing 30 year study of raw fed dogs and cats. You can submit your dog(s) in the project for FREE after you transition. My dogs have been part of the project since 2017)

Let's Connect

Social Media

- Youtube: youtube.com/c/dogdad
- Facebook: www.facebook.com/dogdadofficial/
- Instagram: @dogdadofficial
- Twitter: @dogdadofficial

To Work 1 on 1 With Me:

www.rawfeeding101.com/1on1

RAW FEEDING 1⬤1

Made in the USA
Lexington, KY
17 January 2019

"Raw Feeding should be simple."

Scratching, itching, vomiting, diarrhea yeast-filled ears and paws...these are the problems plaguing today's modern dog. The common culprit? An inappropriate diet The solution? A species appropriate diet of fresh foods.

In this book you will learn:
› How to transition your dog to a fresh food diet
› How to prepare fresh food meals
› How to safely feed raw meaty bones
› Sanitary practices to prevent illness
› Important fresh food information

Scott J. Marshall II "Dog Dad" shares raw feeding content on his YouTube channel. He is the certified raw dog food nutrition specialist behind the Raw Feeding 101 online video course. Scott lives in Utah with his wife and two dogs.

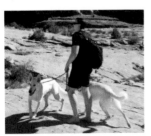

ISBN 9781719246880